About Island Press

Since 1984, the nonprofit organization Island Press has been stimulating, shaping, and communicating ideas that are essential for solving environmental problems worldwide. With more than 800 titles in print and some 40 new releases each year, we are the nation's leading publisher on environmental issues. We identify innovative thinkers and emerging trends in the environmental field. We work with world-renowned experts and authors to develop cross-disciplinary solutions to environmental challenges.

Island Press designs and executes educational campaigns in conjunction with our authors to communicate their critical messages in print, in person, and online using the latest technologies, innovative programs, and the media. Our goal is to reach targeted audiences—scientists, policymakers, environmental advocates, urban planners, the media, and concerned citizens—with information that can be used to create the framework for long-term ecological health and human well-being.

Island Press gratefully acknowledges major support of our work by The Agua Fund, The Andrew W. Mellon Foundation, Betsy & Jesse Fink Foundation, The Bobolink Foundation, The Curtis and Edith Munson Foundation, Forrest C. and Frances H. Lattner Foundation, G.O. Forward Fund of the Saint Paul Foundation, Gordon and Betty Moore Foundation, The Kresge Foundation, The Margaret A. Cargill Foundation, New Mexico Water Initiative, a project of Hanuman Foundation, The Overbrook Foundation, The S.D. Bechtel, Jr. Foundation, The Summit Charitable Foundation, Inc., V. Kann Rasmussen Foundation, The Wallace Alexander Gerbode Foundation, and other generous supporters.

The opinions expressed in this book are those of the author(s) and do not necessarily reflect the views of our supporters.

PUBLIC PRODUCE

Public Produce

Cultivating Our Parks, Plazas,
and Streets for Healthier Cities

Darrin Nordahl

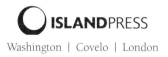

ISLANDPRESS

Washington | Covelo | London

Island Press is a trademark of The Center for Resource Economics.

Library of Congress Cataloging-in-Publication Data

Nordahl, Darrin.
Public produce : cultivating our parks, plazas, and streets for healthier cities /
Darrin Nordahl.
pages cm
Includes bibliographical references and index.
ISBN 978-1-61091-549-6 (pbk. : alk. paper) — ISBN 1-61091-549-6 (pbk. :
alk. paper) — ISBN 978-1-61091-550-2 (ebook) — ISBN 1-61091-550-X
(ebook) 1. Urban agriculture. 2. Urban gardening. 3. City planning—Health
aspects. 4. Streetscapes (Urban design) I. Title.
S441.N76 2014
635.09173'2—dc23
2014008745

♻ Printed on recycled, acid-free paper

Manufactured in the United States of America

10 9 8 7 6 5 4 3 2 1

Keywords: Beacon Food Forest, Berkeley, Calgary, Center for Urban Education
about Sustainable Agriculture, Chicago, community garden, community-
supported agriculture, Detroit, Edible Schoolyard, farmers' market, food desert,
food justice, food literacy, food safety, food security, forage, Kamloops, local
food, Los Angeles, Michael Pollan, New York City, obesity, Portland, Provo,
public health, public policy, public space, Ron Finley, San Francisco, Seattle,
slow food, social equity, transitional gardens, urban agriculture, urban design,
urban farming, Worthington, victory garden

For Lara, Noe, Nate, and Mia
and for Tom Flaherty

Contents

Flashback:
Notes on the Updated Edition

It's 2009. America's economic crisis that tipped two years ago has triggered a global recession. Every month, hundreds of thousand of American workers find themselves out of a job and the unemployment rate climbs above 10 percent. Home prices continue to freefall while gasoline prices creep higher. Food banks across the country report record numbers of folks seeking hunger relief. America's economy is the shakiest it has been since the Great Depression, coercing Congress to pass the American Recovery and Reinvestment Act: an 800-billion-dollar tourniquet to stem the financial bleeding.

An idea emerges from the economic wallows of 2009. *Public Produce* is published, a timely response to the legions of Americans who suddenly have to choose between eating or paying rent. Turning public space into a community horn of plenty could be an effective stimulus package in its own right. But it is only an idea, a nascent strategy to bolster the health and wealth of a society reeling from the Great Recession.

Flash forward five years. Communities are digging out of the financial rubble and public produce is blossoming. Vegetable gardens welcome citizens to city halls from Bainbridge Island to Baltimore. Seattleites are cultivating street medians and Portlanders are gleaning thousands of pounds of apples, plums, and cherries from neighborhood trees. But these civic fruits and vegetables aren't confined to the United States. Across the 49th parallel, Calgary is planting fruit orchards in community parks, and an empty lot in downtown Kamloops, British Columbia, is transformed into a veritable alfresco produce aisle.

What a difference a half decade makes.

When I wrote *Public Produce* in 2009, I was focusing a vision. Someone planted an apple tree in a public park in Berkeley, California, while a homeowner a few blocks over planted a fig tree along the sidewalk. A public official in one Iowa town talked about creating an edible oasis from a decrepit parking lot, while another in Iowa's capital sought to revitalize several blocks of a distressed neighborhood by planting fruit and nut trees. The initiatives were inspiring, and the potential to weave these smaller, isolated efforts into something larger and more cohesive compelled me to write the book. I thought if more civic leaders took up similar food-based initiatives, and implemented them on a larger, more integrated network of urban space, then public produce could help bolster food security and community prosperity amid troubled economic times. The idea was burgeoning in 2009, but there were few concrete examples of action.

Today, things are different. Public produce is no longer just a "Gosh, wouldn't it be nice if we could grow fruits and vegetables for the public to harvest?" idea. Municipalities across the United States and Canada are doing it. And they have been doing it for the last five years. This revised edition profiles those communities and community officials that are rethinking the role of public space in cities, and how our parks, plazas, squares, and streets can sustain health and happiness through fresh produce.

But my focus has also changed. In the first edition of *Public Produce*, I looked at how public space and public policy could work together to reduce food insecurity, primarily for the destitute and perennially hungry. Indeed, when even the middle class began to wonder where their next meal would come from, I felt it was our societal obligation to provide healthy, low-cost food options to those down on their luck.

In the course of five years, I discovered that regardless of our particular economic station, we all benefit from better access to fresh fruits and vegetables. Most people desire to eat healthier and have an innate passion for good food. Most also have an innate passion for nature. We love witnessing plants transform into ripe produce, reminding us food does not originate from the supermarket, but from the soil. And we revel in the wonderment in children's eyes when they pluck an apple off a tree or a carrot from the ground. In other words, offering the opportunity to pick a meal from the park or street median has value to more folks than just the impoverished.

Besides, the food headlines of 2009 have hardly changed five years later. Yes, our pocketbooks are getting fatter; but so are we. Obesity rates continue to balloon in this country, and the epidemic is the focus of many a news story. Pathogen outbreaks, the rising cost of food, and the growing demand for local food options continue to make the front page as well. We as a nation are becoming increasingly concerned with where our food comes from and how it is produced. These frequent exposés have alerted civic leaders to the inextricable bonds between food, community, and our quality of life.

I was also concerned that by focusing heavily on the poor, this concept of growing fruits and vegetables in public space for anyone to harvest would only be embraced by liberals (and even then, only those on the Left Coast). But I needn't have worried. I've learned in the last five years that public produce appeases both party platforms. It is a form of social equity and food justice, and reconnects us to our agrarian past. Seeing fruits and vegetables in the public spaces we pass by daily also teaches us about food, where it comes from, and how to grow it. Many of the public produce programs are rooted in education, teaching us how to be more self-reliant. Public produce is not a government handout, but a life skill to help us get by.

If you haven't read the first edition of *Public Produce*, this new, completely revised version is all you'll need to be inspired by and learn from the pioneering public officials who have implemented fruit and vegetable gardens to correct what many think are intractable problems: food insecurity and our declining health and wealth.

If you *have* read the first edition, first let me say thank you. But let me also say that you will find this update to *Public Produce* even more appetizing. Every chapter has been extensively revised. This is a livelier publication, and the examples I have included in this edition are even more relevant and provocative. The chapter on maintenance and aesthetics (chapter 5) is particularly useful. It has been completely updated, now packed with insights from public officials who have managed public produce gardens for the last five years. I have learned much in the last half decade from these innovative souls, and you will, too.

A Guerilla on Strawberry Street

FOOD IS THE PROBLEM, AND IT IS THE SOLUTION.

This is the salient message Ron Finley shares during his popular TED talk as he details the woes of South Central Los Angeles. It is a neighborhood racked by poverty, racial riots, and turf wars. South Central is home to the Bloods and the Crips, two rival gangs with a penchant for drugs and violence. The infamy of South Central is legendary, spawning Hollywood films such as *Boyz n the Hood* and *Colors*, two flicks that revealed to the world the brutal, abject conditions within this supposed City of Angels. South Central became so notorious that the City of Los Angeles struck its name from the record. South Central is no more, at least according to official city maps. It is now South Los Angeles, a bureaucratic strategy to improve the image of this stigmatized part of town.

But Finley doesn't buy it. To him, it's still the same old South

Central, a place dominated in the public eye by vacant lots, liquor stores, and fast food. Early demise is imminent in the South Central population. But not because of reasons you might expect. Drugs and bullets aren't killing folks in South Central. Food is.

"The drive-thrus are killing more people than the drive-bys," notes Finley. "People are dying from curable diseases in South Central." Like 26.5 million other Americans, Finley lives in a food "desert," a place where fresh, healthy, and affordable food is as scarce as water in the Sahara.[1] Obesity rates in South Central are five times what they are in neighboring Beverly Hills. Finley has to drive forty-five minutes round-trip just to buy organic apples. The lack of access to cheap *and* nutritious food is literally crippling South Central. "I see wheel chairs bought and sold like used cars," laments Finley. "I see dialysis centers popping up like Starbucks. And this has to stop."[2]

In 2010 Finley had had enough. The lack of fresh fruits and vegetables in his neighborhood compelled him to do something radical. After all, desperate times call for desperate measures. Finley became a guerilla gardener.

Finley commandeered the parkway outside his house: a strip of landscape about 150 feet long and 10 feet wide between the sidewalk and curb. He and his volunteer group planted what Finley calls a food forest: "fruit trees, vegetables, the whole nine." What makes Finley's tactics extreme is that he planted his garden on public land without permission from the City. But here's the rub. Even though Finley does not have exclusive rights to this strip of land, he is the one responsible for its upkeep and maintenance. The way Finley sees it, "I can do whatever the hell I want! Since it's my responsibility and I gotta maintain it." And the way Finley decided to maintain it was through fresh produce. "It was beautiful," gushed Finley. But he wasn't speaking about the aesthetics of the garden particularly (though the arrangement was visually stunning). The real beauty was the reason for the fruit and vegetables in the first place. Finley didn't plant produce just for himself, but for anyone passing by—a gift from a concerned individual to his community.

For his incredibly heartfelt display of goodwill, Finley was rewarded by the City of Los Angeles with a citation. Someone complained about the garden, and the City came down on Finley, ordering him to remove his plants. Finley refused. Next came a warrant. Finley was dumbfounded. "C'mon, really? A warrant for planting food on a piece of land [the City] could care less about?"

Finley had a valid point, made more logical when you learn that Los Angeles leads the nation in the amount of vacant parcels owned by a municipality, some twenty-six square miles of land. It is the equivalent of twenty Central Parks, or "enough space to plant 725 million tomato plants," Finley quipped. Yet the City does nothing with this land.

Finley fought back. He drafted a petition and received over nine hundred signatures in support of his public produce garden. The *L.A. Times* ran a story, and contacted Finley's councilman. The councilman then called Finley and declared support for Finley's efforts. "But really, why wouldn't you support this?" Finley asked rhetorically. His food forest didn't just provide his neighbors with fresh food. Finley's fruits had financial value as well. "This is my gospel," Finley preaches. "I'm telling people to grow their own food. Growing your own food is like printing your own money." He's right. One dollar of seed could generate $75 of fresh produce. And in a community where many are out of work and have no idea where their next meal may come from, planting produce in public spaces enriches both body and bank account.

But there's more. Finley has witnessed the transformative effects his garden has had on the neighborhood. "To change the community, you have to change the composition of the soil," Finley says. "And we are the soil. You'd be surprised how kids are affected by this. Gardening is the most therapeutic and defiant act you can do, especially in the inner city. Plus, you get strawberries."

The amount of good this street-side garden gives South Central

—and Finley himself—is obvious. Finley spends a lot of time in his garden, but he enjoys it. He calls himself a street artist, and gardening is Finley's graffiti. His canvas is made of dirt, and his palette is mixed with sunflower yellow, collard green, and strawberry red. It is a masterpiece Finley and the community are quite proud of. But colleagues often ask him, "Fin, aren't you afraid people are going to steal your food?"

Finley just shakes his head. "Hell no, I ain't afraid they're gonna steal it. That's why it's on the street. That's the whole idea."

This book advocates for more Ron Finleys in the world. More specifically, this book examines the great community good that can result simply from planting fruits and vegetables in our public spaces. Maybe you're thinking, "Sounds great! I'm aboard, let's do it!" Or maybe you are hesitant, like the public officials in the City of Los Angeles. Sure, it sounds easy, but maybe you think agriculture doesn't belong in cities. Especially in inner cities. Especially in *public places* in inner cities.

In defense of the bureaucrat, I can understand why so many are reluctant to embrace food grown in public spaces free for the picking. For one, we have become a food dysfunctional society. For a nation founded on agrarian ideals—when crops permeated every nook and cranny of our towns and cities for centuries—it is baffling we would bristle at the thought of fruits and vegetables in parks and plazas, along our streets, and around our civic buildings. Until you understand the great ideological shift in how we Americans produce, and subsequently view, food. That shift—and this story—begins shortly after World War II.

Public opinion of what an American city should be profoundly changed in the late 1940s. The return of our troops spawned an urge for a different kind of settlement, a tweak in the American Dream. A new vision of the American city became manifest with urban renewal, when dense inner cities were gutted, opening up space for freeways, residential towers, and large corporate centers surrounded by expansive concrete plazas. Unfortunately, this new vision didn't include farms, produce stands, or fussy vegetable patches, including those tremendously popular victory gardens that were so essential in bolstering our troops and Allies. Our cities were streamlined and compartmentalized, with the home, workplace, marketplace, and open space all separated from each other. The zoning that mandated the separation of land uses also prohibited agriculture within the more urbanized neighborhoods of the city. Once the land uses were separated and the impurities of agriculture removed, a new settlement was born—one that commanded cleaner landscaping and well-manicured, sterile varieties of trees, shrubs, and groundcovers.

Suburban sprawl picked up where zoning laws left off and pushed agriculture even farther from the city center. Those farms not consumed by residential subdivisions became aggregated with other farms. As such, the second half of the twentieth century saw the number of farms in America dwindle from more than six million in 1940 to just two million at the dawn of the new millennium.[3]

And so, the agricultural paradigm had shifted. The pervasive ideology of the mid-twentieth century became that food production was no longer suitable in and around our cities, as it had been since the emergence of civilization. Growing fruits and vegetables was no longer the work of community-minded individuals and families on small local farms, but endeavors better suited to corporate-owned, factory-like "agribusiness" in more distant parts of the country. And with the disappearance of the ubiquitous small family farms, public gardens, and individual produce markets and stands, we forgot what was previously common knowledge: where food comes from, how it's grown, and when it is ready to eat.

But the pendulum swings. Now, as the twenty-first century is well underway, a cresting wave is readying the backlash against large-scale corporate agriculture on fields hundreds—if not thousands—of miles from where we live; against mass-produced, chemically grown produce; against the rising costs of food and the declining health of the American people. The organic movement is ceding to the "buy-local" movement; fast food is now a pejorative term,[4] while "slow food" seems to be the choice of the future. Farmers' markets, community-supported agriculture groups (CSAs), and small produce stands are part of a burgeoning system of local agriculture that is enjoying a popularity not witnessed in more than half a century. And the time is ripe to explore how we can expand this network of local food options to meet the growing demand of consumers by bringing agriculture back into our cities.

This book explores how to make agriculture the apple in the public eye once again, by giving city dwellers a bounty of options for gathering food from the urban environment. Of course, I'm not suggesting we banish our current system of agriculture; at least not entirely. It is unrealistic to believe Americans will want to return to subsistence agriculture. It is equally absurd to assume we will desire to eat only locally grown, seasonally available produce. We will still want bananas, oranges, and avocados even if we live in Wisconsin, or tomatoes, peppers, and corn in February, regardless of where we live. This book is about providing food choices within the city—where the majority of the US population lives today (and with continued urbanization projected)—and about how to achieve healthful, low-cost supplements to our diet. *Public Produce* examines local food options through the lens of social equity: closing the food gap between the inner-city poor (and increasingly the lower-middle and middle class) and the high prices of supermarket organic and farmers' market produce; improving the health of the American population, especially our children, who increasingly lack everyday accessibility to fresh produce; providing a sense of self-sufficiency to even the well-to-do by giving them an opportunity to forage for ripe fruits and vegetables; and recognizing the social relationships and prosperous citizenry that could result if city spaces could help provide food for all.

Toward the goal of food justice, this book is specifically about fresh produce grown on public land and thus available to all members of the public—for gathering or gleaning, for purchase or trade. And, because this food is grown on public land, this book examines the efforts, programs, and policies that are being ushered and implemented by local governments. If a network of locally available, publicly accessible produce is to be successful, the largest single landowner within the city—the municipality itself—will have to be engaged.

At the heart of these pleas for a more equitable system of food production is *food security*: daily access to an adequate supply of nutritious, affordable, and safe food. The frequent outbreaks of *Escherichia coli* (*E. coli*) infecting spinach from California and clover sprouts from Jimmy John's, along with *Salmonella* contaminating peppers packed in Texas, peanuts in Georgia, and pistachios in California, reveal that our fresh-produce farms and distribution centers may not be as safe and sterile as we thought. Climate change, which is producing drought in California, freezing temperatures in Florida, and floods in Iowa, is reducing crop yields. Pest infestations are reducing crop yields as well. Florida Department of Agriculture spokesman Terence McElroy notes, "Our office is getting reports of at least one new pest or disease of significant economic concern per month."[5] Ordinarily, a pest outbreak in Florida (or Iowa or California) shouldn't be cause for too much concern for the rest of the country. But when only a couple of states provide the overwhelming bulk of our fresh fruits, vegetables, nuts, and grains, a local infestation can have national consequences. It is unfortunate that relatively isolated agricultural problems in a couple of states are felt nationwide, but such is the nature of our current food-supply system. As a measure of insurance, this is perhaps reason enough to employ a more local, public system of food production.

Weather anomalies, pest infestations, and bacterial contaminations obviously limit the food supply, which in turn drives up prices. But there is another, more pervasive reason for the recent spike in the cost of fresh produce: oil. The large-scale, specialized agribusinesses that furnish much of the food in the United States rely heavily on oil. Idaho produces much of the nation's potatoes; Washington, our apples; Michigan, our blueberries; California, our broccoli; and Iowa, our corn and soybeans (the bulk of which is consumed by livestock, or processed into corn syrup, ethanol, and partially hydrogenated oils or trans fats). The soaring cost of oil affects these large-scale agricultural endeavors in many interconnected ways: from the fuel used to power the tractors and combine harvesters; to the petroleum-based herbicides and pesticides liberally sprayed on the fields; and back to the fuel used to power the diesel trucks that deliver the produce hundreds, if not thousands, of miles to our urban markets.

That increasing distance to market—measured in "food miles"—is of great concern in the face of a shrinking oil supply and its ever-rising cost. If our produce only came from within our nation's boundaries, perhaps those food miles could be manageable. We now import considerable produce from large, multinational food conglomerates in Canada, Mexico, Chile, and increasingly, New Zealand and China. As it is, the average produce item in our supermarkets comes from more than 1,500 miles away.[6] As food producers become bigger and more specialized, their distances away from cities become greater, and energy consumption increases. Reduce the distance an apple travels from the tree to your hand, and a reduction in price could result.

The people most affected by the rising cost of produce are low-income individuals, as well as single-parent and single-income families. Foodborne pathogens and pests, on the other hand, affect everyone, regardless of financial position, and have become a national security concern. Hunger is obviously the result of food insecurity and can be seen the world over. But in America, obesity is a food security issue as well. The farmer is no match for the deep-pocket marketing campaigns of our fast-food chains and processed-food conglomerates, especially during tough economic times. (Even amidst the Great Recession, McDonald's posted strong earnings.)[7] Children are especially susceptible to advertising, a fact marketing consultants use to their advantage. To combat the salvo of fast-food and processed-food commercials, signs, and billboard advertisements, fresh, whole foods ought to be equally omnipresent in our urban environment, to remind children—everyone, for that matter—of healthful food alternatives. We thus have to change the way we think about plants and public spaces in the urban environment—not as providing merely aesthetic and recreational value but sustenance and nutrition as well.

Addressing food security is reason enough to explore the notion of a more public system of food production, but there are certainly more. As will become evident in subsequent chapters, public produce is helping to attain broad civic aims, such as providing small-business financial assistance; boosting civic pride and building community; reducing crime; strengthening our connection to place; and reintroducing seasons and the natural cycles of life to our young and not-so-young. In short, food choices found in our urban surrounds can give citizens a more bountiful life.

There are also environmental benefits. Former Chicago mayor Richard M. Daley led the way in creating a more environmentally friendly city through the greening of his city's public spaces. Chicago offers an inspirational success story, rocketing from what many people thought was a fallen, dilapidated city to one of the greenest and greatest cities in the nation. Daley's investment in the environment not only has improved the ecology and aesthetics of Chicago but has brought in billions of tourist dollars, triggered a spike in development interest, and garnered the attention of civic leaders and city builders around the globe.

The physical greening of Chicago—through the planting of countless trees, shrubs, and perennials along the streets, atop roofs, and within parks, plazas, and other public spaces of Chicago— is certainly praiseworthy. However, the next evolution of greening our civic spaces should focus on the value each tree, shrub, and perennial provides to the public. An elm tree, for example, offers beauty and shade, providing a natural, fossil-free source of air conditioning. It also sequesters carbon dioxide emissions and replaces them with oxygen; creates habitat for birds and other urban wildlife; and reduces stormwater runoff. An elm tree also helps give scale and interest to the street, enhances buildings, and as such, raises property values. But can a tree do all of these things and go one step further, by providing food for human consumption as well? Adding food to the list of benefits a public tree can provide greatly increases its value to the city's citizens and visitors. Landscape architects, as designers of our urban public spaces, have proven adept at using plants to address concerns of comfort, maintenance, aesthetics, and other socio-environmental factors. Adding food to that list is well within their regimen, and something that should be demanded by clients.

The best place to realize the environmental, economic, and equitable benefits of a more local system of agriculture may not be in some rural or exurban location, but in and among the places we pass by daily on our way to work, home, school, commerce, and recreation. It may not seem so to the casual observer, but when the sum of all the public spaces in a typical city is figured, the municipality itself is the largest single landlord. The sheer abundance of land within public control necessitates a hard look at how it can best serve the needs of its shareholders. This could mean the land needs to be as productive as biologically possible, that every square foot has value to those who use it or pass by. Plazas, parks, town squares, city streets, and the grounds around our parking lots, libraries, schools, city halls, and courthouses are prime locations to consider when rethinking the role of public space in our cities—and how to add value to those spaces if they are currently underutilized. Hence, the efforts profiled in this book go beyond the mere greening of our city spaces; they illustrate how public space can produce a commodity that can be consumed by the human end user, namely, food.

More than just providing places for the occasional community garden, the intent of this book is to examine how the intricate web of public space within cities can be used for more prolific food production. This is a critical examination of *all* the plants in *all* the public spaces within the city: fruit trees and shrubs along streets and in medians; orchards in parks; herbs and vegetables in planters located on plazas and sidewalks in our commercial areas; and rooftop agriculture, to name a few. Most notably, this book scrutinizes the dense, multistranded network of food-growing opportunities accessible to the public that could be realized with the active support and involvement of city government.

Some government officials already recognize the dire need for municipalities to engage in food-producing alternatives. Susan Anderson, former chief of horticulture for the City of Davenport, Iowa, argues that one responsibility of local government "falls in the area of dedication of land and management of it for the common good. In an urban environment how do we provide the opportunity for people to access land they can use for food?" Anderson uses her home city of Davenport as an example: "We are an urban community. Preserving agricultural land as a resource is important but in an urban setting commercial, large-scale farming operations of the Midwest variety aren't going to help someone downtown."

Anderson believes local government should set aside public land expressly for the purpose of urban gardening. She further contends that such land dedication and management "becomes a wellness issue for the community. Actually, it is very attractive to those of us who are concerned with the quality of our soils, depletion of minerals and nutrients essential to healthy people and plants, to see a community that provides access to locally grown, fresh food sources and/or the ability to create our own."[8]

The system of municipal agriculture that Anderson describes could be a manifestation of what the late Thomas Lyson, a distinguished professor in the Department of Development Sociology at Cornell University, called "civic agriculture." According to Lyson, civic agriculture "embodies a commitment to developing and strengthening an economically, environmentally, and socially sustainable system of agriculture and food production that relies on local resources and serves local markets and consumers. The imperative to earn a profit is filtered through a set of cooperative and mutually supporting social relations. Community problem solving rather than individual competition is the foundation of civic agriculture."

By contrast, Lyson argued, "Large-scale, absentee-owned, factory-like fruit and vegetable farms that rely on large numbers of migrant workers and sell their produce for export around the world would not be deemed very civic."[9]

Lyson recognized a growing hunger for civic agriculture, as evidenced by the popularity of farmers' markets, CSAs, and community gardens throughout the country. Farmers' markets increased from 1,750 in 1994 to nearly 8,200 today. CSAs were virtually non-existent a couple of decades ago. In 1986, there were just two. Now there are more than 6,000.[10] The slow-food movement is garnering interest throughout the country. The term *locavore* now appears in *The New Oxford American Dictionary*; it means someone who only eats what is grown or produced locally, usually within a hundred mile radius.[11] Eating only that food which is produced within 100 miles of your dinner plate is an admirable challenge given today's methods of food production, but it is a distance that would seem formidably long to our grandparents and great-grandparents. For them, the thought of carrots, tomatoes, onions, or potatoes traveling 100 miles to consumers would be unfathomable.

In addition to advocating for smaller, independent farms located closer to cities, planners, environmentalists, policy makers, and educators are also urging the preservation of existing agricultural land within the city boundary, and, in some cases, new farms interwoven into the urban fabric. Unfortunately, it may be too late for this latter policy reform in some cities. Some metropolises are just too big to have farms very near the principal city's center. For those older, denser cities along the Mid-Atlantic, for example, there is little to no agricultural land left within or around the city to preserve;

and little room for new farms. Nor would this policy benefit inner-city or downtown residents in most urban communities, as Susan Anderson noted. For these communities, the only option for local food production may be to explore the available, arable public land within their urban environs as an opportunity to establish a vast network of small-scale, yet abundant food-producing activities.

Of course, many hurdles lie in the way of providing a healthier, more equitable urban landscape. One of the tallest may be our newly gained ignorance of food. We as a nation will have to re-educate ourselves about food, what it looks like, where it grows, and when it is ready to harvest. In short, we need to get back to our agrarian roots. I have witnessed adults convinced that pineapples grow on trees. A very young, very naïve vegan acquaintance once explained she could not have coconut milk because she gave up meat and dairy in her diet. I have been a member of a well-intentioned CSA that did not know the proper time to harvest okra. What were delivered were large pods the size of Anaheim chili peppers. (When okra pods are allowed to grow large, their flesh becomes woody, rendering them inedible.)

Even people living in rural areas are no more food-savvy than the typical big-city dweller; ironically, less so. I worked with a young woman from rural Iowa who had never tasted eggplant, and admitted she probably would not be able to recognize one. (Eggplant, incidentally, grows quite well in Iowa.) My neighbor recounted a conversation she had with a teenager who loved to eat guacamole, but had never seen an avocado. Many Iowans never have eaten tofu, tasted soy milk, or ever heard of edamame—yet Iowa is the largest grower of soybeans in the country. On a recent educational tour of Davenport's conservatory that was aimed at teaching children about food and plants, one child asked if the sunflowers would grow "ranch-flavored" seeds. Another asked if the small oranges on a tree in the grow house were pumpkins or watermelons. As Susan Anderson lamented, "Do you think kids in Iowa know where their food comes from? These kids live in

Davenport, not Chicago. They can drive five miles and see a farm. On a good day they can smell the corn-processing plants. There is a huge disconnect going on. Unless we work to initiate a process for change it won't get better."[12]

If public produce is to succeed in our cities, educational programs are needed to reacquaint us with food, to help us recognize which plants are edible and which are ornamental, and to teach us how to plant, how to care for, and how to harvest food. We have much to relearn about food and agriculture as we explore opportunities for them in our urban settings.

Thankfully, we can learn from the various bits of municipally organized urban agriculture on public land that are already happening across the country. This book highlights a few of those efforts. Many of these efforts are, admittedly, small in scope. Collectively, they indicate a budding shift in public policy taking root throughout the country. Urban agriculture on public land, though currently in an embryonic state, is certainly real. The collection of assorted, independent examples underway throughout North American cities big and small offers a glimpse of a trend driven not by a central government policy, but by a local one, and the communities' desire for more economically viable, environmentally sustainable, locally available, and healthful choices in food production. These efforts are varied: restaurateurs seeking to reduce overhead costs by foraging for their own produce, or willing to trade for it; city officials, both hired and elected, using public space under their management for the production of food; school grounds being replanted with edible gardens to help teach children where food comes from and how to grow it (and to entice them to eat healthier); neighborhood groups gleaning from urban fruit trees and promoting usufruct laws (the legal right to harvest fruit belonging to a private party if it overhangs, or is accessible from, public property); and the rise of guerilla gardeners like Ron Finley—vigilantes who take over vacant or blighted land in the city and return it to productivity and beauty through the planting and management of gardens.

Though their work is benign and their mission inspirational, there is reason for their "guerrilla" moniker: their tactics border on extremism. Regardless, their actions and the others mentioned point out the lengths to which citizens are going to increase accessibility of fresh produce.

It is time for municipal government to recognize these urban food-producing endeavors, embrace them, help manage them, and even build upon them. Indeed, many of the grassroots efforts are initiated by government employees themselves—dedicated civil servants bent on improving the quality of the city and the quality of life of the city's inhabitants. Their efforts illustrate both a need and a desire to supplement our existing food-production methods outside the city with opportunities within the city itself. Working in concert, each venture—regardless of size or scope—contributes to making fresh produce more available to the public. And, in so doing, each can help reinforce a sense of place and build community, nourish the needy, provide economic assistance to entrepreneurs, promote food literacy and good health to all, and return a bit of agrarianism back into our urbanism.

Chapter 1

Food Security

I'M SITTING ON THE BACK PATIO OF A CAFÉ IN SACRAMENTO, California, and all everyone is talking about is the gorgeous weather: sunny and warm, with a perfect springtime temperature of 79 degrees. Except it is not springtime. It is the dead of winter, and 79 degrees is the warmest temperature ever recorded in Sacramento in January. Not by 1 degree or 2 degrees, but by 5. In fact, today is the tenth day this month Sacramento has posted record high temperatures.

Now, maybe a hotter-than-ever January isn't worth getting too worried over. After all, Californians do not typically feel any guilt basking in unseasonably warm weather, even when the rest of the nation is being flash-frozen by the historic polar vortex of 2014. But this record-shattering warm spell is different, because it comes on the heels of the driest year ever recorded in the state. "We're facing perhaps the worst drought that California has ever seen since records began being kept about 100 years ago," noted Governor Jerry Brown during a press conference to declare a drought emergency.[1]

Some scientists believe the drought is even rarer. B. Lynn Ingram, a paleoclimatologist at UC Berkeley, is able to discern wet years from dry ones in California—even before records were kept—simply by examining the annual growth rings of trees. Wide rings indicate lots of growth, thanks to ample rainfall. In dry years, trees hardly enlarge, reflected by a very narrow band. The state's native redwoods, sequoias, and bristlecone pines provide Ingram with weather data that go back centuries.

So what do the trees say to Ingram? This latest drought might be the worst since Sir Francis Drake visited California in 1580.[2]

At his press conference, Governor Brown didn't blame the record temperatures or aridity on climate change. Even climatologists aren't sure if the abnormal weather is the result of man or Mother Nature's capriciousness. But the fact is, these anomalies are becoming more regular in California. In 2008, after what was then the driest spring in eighty-eight years, Governor Schwarzenegger declared a drought emergency as well. That's two emergency declarations in six years. These may not be aberrations after all. Some scientists speculate the west is witnessing the beginning of a mega-drought— severely dry conditions that last for decades. California's recent spate of hot winter days and parched soils could be, as Governor Brown forecasted, "a stark warning of things to come."[3]

If Governor Brown's ominous prediction proves prescient, everyone in America should be deeply concerned. Why? Because California produces 95 percent of the nation's broccoli, that's why. The state also grows 86 percent of our domestic cauliflower, 98 percent of garlic, 94 percent of celery, 97 percent of plums, 95 percent of nectarines, and 100 percent of clingstone peaches. Those bright red luscious strawberries that we love to eat plain or drizzled in chocolate? Ninety-two percent of them come from California. And don't forget those healthy leafy greens. California is the Salad Bowl

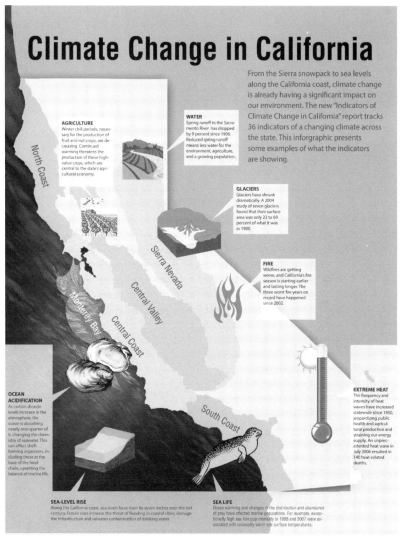

Climate Change in California

From the Sierra snowpack to sea levels along the California coast, climate change is already having a significant impact on our environment. The new "Indicators of Climate Change in California" report tracks 36 indicators of a changing climate across the state. This inforgraphic presents some examples of what the indicators are showing.

AGRICULTURE
Winter chill periods, necessary for the production of fruit and nut crops, are decreasing. Continued warming threatens the production of these high-value crops, which are central to the state's agricultural economy.

WATER
Spring runoff to the Sacramento River has dropped by 9 percent since 1906. Reduced spring runoff means less water for the environment, agriculture, and a growing population.

GLACIERS
Glaciers have shrunk dramatically. A 2004 study of seven glaciers found that their surface area was only 22 to 69 percent of what it was in 1900.

FIRE
Wildfires are getting worse, and California's fire season is starting earlier and lasting longer. The three worst fire years on record have happened since 2002.

OCEAN ACIDIFICATION
As carbon dioxide levels increase in the atmosphere, the ocean is absorbing nearly one-quarter of it, changing the chemistry of seawater. This can affect shell-forming organisms, including those at the base of the food chain, upsetting the balance of marine life.

EXTREME HEAT
The frequency and intensity of heat waves have increased statewide since 1950, jeopardizing public health and agricultural production and straining our energy supply. An unprecedented heat wave in July 2006 resulted in 140 heat-related deaths.

North Coast

Sierra Nevada

Central Valley

Monterey Bay

Central Coast

South Coast

SEA-LEVEL RISE
Along the California coast, sea levels have risen by seven inches over the last century. Future rises increase the threat of flooding in coastal cities, damage the infrastructure and saltwater contamination of drinking water.

SEA LIFE
Ocean warming and changes in the distribution and abundance of prey have affected marine populations. For example, exceptionally high sea lion pup mortality in 1998 and 2007 were associated with unusually warm sea surface temperatures.

Change in California's climate is profoundly impacting ecology as well as agriculture. (Office of Environmental Health Hazard Assessment, California Environmental Protection Agency. Indicators of Climate Change in California, August 2013. Available online at http://www.oehha.ca.gov/multimedia/epic/2013EnvIndicatorReport .html.)

of the United States, producing 85 percent of the nation's leaf lettuce and spinach.

California is also the primary grower of tree nuts, supplying 99 percent of our country's walnuts, almonds, and pistachios. In fact, California is number one in agricultural cash receipts, besting second-ranked Iowa by a whopping 40 percent. *Half* of all the US-grown fruits, vegetables, and nuts come from the Golden State. Regardless of where you live in the country, when you eat produce from your supermarket, you are eating from California.[4]

But here's the hitch. While California has proved to be fertile ground for an appetizing array of fruits, vegetables, and nuts, higher temperatures and receding rainfall won't just curtail yields, it could obliterate California's ability to feed the nation. Such is the precarious nature of our current food supply system.

It wasn't always like this. Not long ago, our decentralized system of agriculture was regarded as the most productive in the world.[5] Millions of smaller farms spread all over the land meant bad weather in one state wasn't bad news for an entire country. Decentralization was our food safety net. We had built into our agricultural supply what engineers would call *redundancy*: the duplication of critical components in a system for the purpose of increasing reliability.

With today's centralized system of agriculture, however, we've put all our eggplants in one basket. And when 300 million people rely on food from just a couple of locations—like California, or Iowa—local weather troubles create catastrophe for the entire country. One or two years of fidgety weather raises food prices, which is concerning enough. But prolonged fits could mean the most prosperous nation in the world goes hungry.

An uncertain climate isn't the only threat to our food prosperity. In fact, food prices have been escalating for over a decade, at a pace far faster than the increases in the cost of living.[6] Sure, Mother Nature has been responsible for rising food costs in some years, such as 2008 when torrential rains flooded millions of acres of corn in Iowa.[7] But the principle reasons for the rise in food costs are tied to production, processing, packaging, and transportation—which are all tied to oil.[8]

In an open letter to the 2008 US president-elect Barack Obama, food expert and best-selling author Michael Pollan outlined just how our current system of food production is compromising not only the American dinner table, but national security. Pollan argues that our complete reliance on fossil fuels for food production spells imminent catastrophe as the era of cheap, abundant, and nonrenewable energy comes to a close. His arguments deftly illustrate the escalating futility of conventional agriculture. Pollan notes that in 1940, 1 calorie of fossil fuel energy produced 2.3 calories of food energy. But with today's industrial system of agriculture, the ratio has flipped to an inefficient, unsustainable equation, as it takes 10 calories of fossil-fuel energy to produce just 1 calorie of modern supermarket food. Pollan maintains that the solution "could not be simpler: we need to wean the American food system off its heavy twentieth-century diet of fossil fuel and put it back on a diet of contemporary sunshine." He advocates for smaller agricultural efforts in more places across the country, "not as a matter of nostalgia for the agrarian past but as a matter of national security." Pollan further contends that "nations that lose the ability to substantially feed themselves will find themselves as gravely compromised in their international dealings as nations that depend on foreign sources of oil presently do. But while there are alternatives to oil, there are no alternatives to food."[9]

Pollan is not alone in his pessimistic views of our current state of food production. James Howard Kunstler, author of *The Long Emergency: Surviving the End of Oil, Climate Change, and Other Converging Catastrophes of the Twenty-First Century*, is also a believer of the decimation that will ultimately result if we do not wean ourselves off of our high-petroleum diet. Many of Kunstler's arguments parallel Pollan's. Kunstler paints a chilling tale of doom for urban

America that is quite frightening—frightening because his predictions do not seem particularly far-fetched. He predicts that smaller communities surrounded by agriculture have the highest hopes of surviving the Long Emergency. He is not so confident about the big cities, however, because they are growing in an unsustainable manner and they haven't had the urge to create or preserve an agricultural belt surrounding them. Kunstler concludes with a realization that our cities cannot continue to grow in the ways that they currently have, and predicts Americans will need to return to some form of agrarian life:

> To put it simply, Americans have been eating oil and natural gas for the past century, at an ever-accelerating pace. Without the massive "inputs" of cheap gasoline and diesel fuel for machines, irrigation, and trucking, or petroleum-based herbicides and pesticides, or fertilizers made out of natural gas, Americans will be compelled to radically reorganize the way food is produced, or starve.[10]

Before we discount Kunstler's and Pollan's arguments as apocalyptic hyperbole, let's recall the many government-guided, community-implemented food production programs in this country that arose from national crises. The most significant—and prolific—of these were the victory gardens of World War II: Twenty million small gardens supplied 40 percent of the fresh vegetables consumed in America.[11] But there were similar food-producing efforts during World War I, the Great Depression, and the Long Depression of the 1890s. During each of these distressed times, amid threats to national security, the federal government rallied the American people around food production, and created programs to educate citizens and assist them in exploiting food-growing opportunities throughout their urban communities.

The agriculture and gardening efforts during those periods of crisis were initiated to help secure our food supply, and the government looked to urban means of food production to supplement the rural farms that were unable to keep up with domestic demand. During World War I, the community agricultural efforts not only stabilized our nation's food supply, but bolstered that of the Allies as well. But more than a food source, the community agriculture efforts, especially the victory gardens, were meant to counteract a host of societal ills associated with crisis by providing "nutritional, psychological, and social returns for the individual and family."[12] These agricultural activities provided work relief for the unemployed; allowed the otherwise helpless women, children, and elderly to participate in the war efforts, giving them a sense of patriotic self-sacrifice; and even provided a form of recreation, allowing people to escape, if only momentarily, the troubles of the times.

Today, the need for similar public agriculture efforts could not be greater. In addition to the concerns that our earlier community food-producing efforts addressed, our current food system has far-reaching environmental and societal health ramifications. What is at stake is threefold: the rising cost of produce (and the resultant effect on our pocketbook); the degradation of our environment; and the declining health of our citizens associated with the obesity epidemic. The gardening and agriculture endeavors during our previous economic depressions and world wars helped supplement the nation's food supply and sustain the American population through periods of food shortages. The great irony today is that the call for more abundant, locally led, and community-organized forms of agriculture is an appeal not so much to supplement our current system of food production as to save us from it.

At the crux of both Pollan's and Kunstler's arguments is our nation's reliance on oil for the production of food. From before the advent of agriculture until the Industrial Revolution, societies never had to rely on fossil fuels to feed themselves. Today, the conventional system of agriculture in the United States relies on fossil fuels for almost every phase of food production: in the manufacturing of fertilizers, pesticides, and herbicides; for powering the complex machinery necessary for tilling, planting, harvesting, washing, sorting, and processing; and in transporting the final food product thousands of miles to our supermarkets. As the bounty of cheap oil dwindles, so too, does our bounty of food. The health of the people, and our environment, will rely on restructuring how food is grown and delivered to the hundreds of millions of people living in our urban environments. Smaller, localized agricultural efforts that do not rely on big, complex machinery, industrial agrichemicals, and vast systems of transport are needed in and around our cities. Fortunately, we already have an abundance of underutilized land within our communities—under public control—that can begin to return the agrarianism that Pollan and Kunstler contend is necessary for survival. Agrarianism and urbanism needn't be mutually exclusive.

Our centralized system of agriculture is eroding not only our environment and economy but our gustatory experience as well, erasing opportunities to enjoy fresh, fully ripened produce. Nonagenarian Juanita Kakalec reflects fondly on the times she used to pick fruit near her home in Washington, DC. "It was just like milking a cow," she reminisced, recalling the simple pleasures of harvesting blueberries fresh from the bush, just a few miles north of the city, in Maryland. "You'd set your bucket down on the ground and just work your fingers over the branches, letting blueberries fall into the pail." Juanita also remembers picking strawberries, as well as visiting the peach and apple orchards in the area.

After her move to North Carolina, Juanita was looking forward to some local peaches. Though not as famous as their Georgian siblings farther south, peaches grown in the Carolinas are wonderfully fragrant, juicy, and tasty. "Unfortunately, you can't find Carolina peaches here in the supermarkets of Carolina," lamented Juanita. "And when you do, they are not very good, because they pick them too early. It seems all the produce these days either comes from California or Peru."[13] (Chile is the likeliest South American source, but her point is valid.)

Whether it is apples, avocados, or asparagus, the globalization of agriculture has given us year-round convenience. But when tied to the rising costs for oil, this convenience comes at a price. It raises the cost of produce and yields a diminished gustatory experience. It is a simple fact: pickers have to harvest fruit before it is ripe so it can be shipped around the world without spoiling. Once the produce has been delivered, it is often gassed with ethylene to induce ripening. Global agriculture also favors cultivated varieties that pack tighter and bruise less, sacrificing flavor and suppleness. The flavor, texture, aroma, and feel of a peach that is harvested early, transported thousands of miles, artificially ripened, then set on a supermarket shelf is quite different from one naturally ripened on the tree and plucked straight from the branch.

Juanita's desire for a fresh, local peach reminded me of an essay written by the provocative New Urbanist architect Daniel Solomon. Aptly titled "Peaches," the essay relays the profound experiences fresh produce provide to the urban dweller. Solomon notes that "food and urbanism are both fundamental to human experience." His argument is that the lack of everyday contact with fresh food in the modern city erodes our sense of place, disconnects us from the natural environment, and threatens an experience that was once commonplace. Solomon writes:

> Foodies worry that masses of people will go through life and never taste a peach that tastes like a peach. The people will survive somehow—it's *peachiness* that is threatened with extinction. In the contemporary world, retaining the full-blown potential of the flavor of a peach as a part of most people's life experience is no small matter. It involves land use policy, banking, union agreements, transportation, and distribution networks as much as it involves peach breeding, which itself is a more complex subject than ever before. In an agrarian society, where the peach trees are outside one's door, the perfect peach is commonplace. Delivering perfect peaches to the modern metropolis is another question.[14]

The land-use policies, transportation, and distribution networks that threaten our quest for perfect produce also threaten our pocketbook. Mark Winne, author of *Closing the Food Gap*, notes that the northeast region of the United States is especially susceptible. New England, at the extremity of both the national transportation system and the food chain, sees substantial increases in food costs compared to California, for example, where much of the country's fresh produce originates. As Winne contends, "The high energy costs associated with shipping food from those regions (near the beginning of the food chain) to New England increase food costs there by 6 to 10 percent."[15]

The distribution and transportation networks are not much shorter for communities in America's Heartland. According to *Food, Fuel, and Freeways*, a report by the Leopold Center for Sustainable Agriculture, the average produce item trucked to a terminal market in Chicago travels more than 1,500 miles. Grapes, broccoli, cauliflower, lettuce, green peas, and spinach all travel over 2,000 miles to reach the Windy City. Most disheartening was the statistic for sweet corn. For Chicagoans, residents of the second-largest corn-producing state in the nation, sweet corn travels, on average, 813 miles to reach them.[16]

As states have become more specialized in agricultural production, citizen access to locally available food has drastically diminished, erasing a bit of cultural heritage in the process. Take Iowa apples, for instance—a fruit with a long history in the Hawkeye State. The first recorded apple orchard in Iowa was planted in 1799, on the banks of the Mississippi River in Lee County.[17] By 1870, apple orchards flourished, and almost 100 percent of the apples consumed in the state were grown in Iowa. By 1925, apple production declined substantially, and Iowa produced just half of the apples consumed there. At the close of the twentieth century, apple production had all but disappeared: only 15 percent of the apples consumed by Iowans were grown in their home state. Now, it is not just apples; almost all of Iowa's fresh-produce supply is

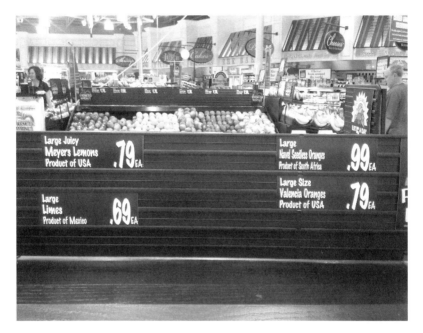

This supermarket citrus stand hints at our global system of agriculture, and the sheer distance that much of our produce has to travel to reach consumers.

produced in other states and trucked in. It is estimated that less than 10 percent of the produce consumed in Iowa is grown in Iowa.[18] In 2007, fresh fruits, nuts, and vegetables represented just 0.13 percent of the state's cash receipts for all of Iowa's agricultural commodities (including livestock). Today, mink pelts produce three times the cash receipts as the state's apple crop.[19]

The specialization of conventional agriculture and its reliance on fossil fuels, coupled with water scarcity in California and weather anomalies across the United States, are complex yet intertwined factors that contribute to the rising cost of food in this country. As if these were not reason enough for Americans to be wary of our current food production and distribution methods, there is yet another cause for concern: food safety. Foodborne illnesses result- ing from pathogen-contaminated food are occurring with alarming regularity in this country, with the most widespread outbreaks happening in recent years. The pathogens most responsible for these food outbreaks are bacteria, specifically *E. coli* O157:H7 and various serotypes of *Salmonella*. Contaminations from these bacteria are typically associated with undercooked meat and eggs, though these pathogens are increasingly finding their way onto our fresh produce as well.

In response to the growing caseload of foodborne illnesses from fresh produce, the US Food and Drug Administration (FDA) drafted the Produce Safety Action Plan. Initiated in 2004, the Action Plan outlines objectives and strategies to prevent contamination from pathogens and to minimize the public health impact when contamination occurs.[20] Even with the Action Plan in place, the FDA is finding it difficult to eradicate pathogen-infected produce and minimize the contamination's spread. Less than two years after the Produce Safety Action Plan was initiated, and in the face of recurring outbreaks of *E. coli* O157:H7 in fresh lettuce, the FDA drafted the Lettuce Safety Initiative. This initiative was aimed primarily at the California lettuce industry, and it sought to assess, document, and potentially regulate industry practices that demonstrated a risk of contaminating the lettuce crop.[21]

At the time the Lettuce Safety Initiative was published, *E. coli* O157:H7–contaminated spinach was beginning to infect people across the country. Over the course of two months, the pathogen-plagued produce sickened almost 200 people from twenty-six states. Three people died from the outbreak. Two were elderly, and the other was a two-year-old child.[22] In the wake of yet another widespread and lethal microbial catastrophe, the FDA's Lettuce Safety Initiative became the Leafy Greens Safety Initiative, and included a broader range of leafy vegetables, including spinach.[23]

In the summer of 2008, the Great Salsa Scare sent consumers of tomatoes and peppers into a panic when it was believed that *Salmonella saintpaul*, previously considered a rare strain of the bacterium, was infecting people who had eaten fresh salsa (e.g., pico de gallo)

from some Tex-Mex restaurants. At first, the outbreak seemed confined to Texas and New Mexico. But in the ensuing weeks, people
across the country became sickened by *S. saintpaul*. When the reports of infections finally ceased in August, four months after the
first infections were documented, the *Salmonella*-tainted produce
had sickened 1,442 people in forty-three states, the District of Columbia, and Canada. The Centers for Disease Control and Prevention (CDC) noted it was the largest outbreak of food-borne illness
in the United States in the past decade.[24]

Not even a month had passed since that infamous record was set
when people became sickened by another serotype of *Salmonella*.
This time, *Salmonella typhimurium* had contaminated peanuts processed by Peanut Corporation of America (PCA) at one of its plants
in Blakely, Georgia. More than thirty million pounds of peanut products were recalled from stores, institutions, and even grade schools
throughout the country, but not before significant health damage
was wrought. From the first cases reported in September 2008 to
April 2009, over 700 people were sickened across forty-six states.
Nine of those people died.[25] Most unsettling, Stewart Parnell, the
owner of PCA, knowingly distributed *Salmonella*-contaminated
products. An FDA report submitted to the US House of Representatives subcommittee investigating the outbreak noted that *Salmonella*
was discovered in PCA's products a dozen different times dating back
to June 2007. In 2006, an audit performed by Nestlé USA at PCA's
Plainview, Texas, facility discovered fifty mouse carcasses in and
around the plant, and a dead pigeon "lying on the ground near the
peanut-receiving door."[26] The FDA report reveals that even though
Parnell was notified by laboratories that his peanut products tested
positive for *Salmonella*, he sold them anyway. "What is virtually unheard of," testified Charles Deibel, president of Deibel Laboratories
Inc., one of the companies that tested PCA products for the Georgia
facility and found *Salmonella*, "is for an entity to disregard those results and place potentially contaminated products into the stream
of commerce." Even up until January 2009, after the *S. typhimurium*

outbreak was linked to peanut butter and peanut paste produced by PCA, Parnell pleaded with FDA officials that his workers "desperately at least need to turn the raw peanuts on our floor into money."[27]

In February of 2009, while illnesses from *S. typhimurium* were still being reported, *S. saintpaul* returned, this time contaminating alfalfa sprouts. More than 200 people across fourteen states were sickened from eating tainted alfalfa. Thankfully, no deaths were reported. In 2012, *E. coli* infected a dozen-and-a-half folks who ate clover sprouts served at Jimmy John's restaurants.[28] *Salmonella*-contaminated pistachios, cucumbers, cantaloupe, and mangoes sickened folks from 2009 to 2013.[29] With these frequent and frightening outbreaks comes an obvious uncertainty and general lack of confidence among Americans with regard to the security of our current food supply and distribution system. An Associated Press–Ipsos poll, conducted during the height of the *S. saintpaul* outbreak, found that almost half of adult Americans fear they may get sick from eating contaminated food. The uneasiness is more apparent with women and minorities. Only one in four women feel "very confident" about the safety of the food they buy. The most fearful group seems to be Hispanics. Half of the Hispanics polled had "little" or "no confidence" in the safety of the food they purchase.[30]

One strategy to help contain future outbreaks and boost consumer confidence is to require labeling that allows produce to be tracked from the dinner plate back to the farm, through the various retailers, processors, distributors, and packers. The lack of such a tracking system is why health officials in the country had a difficult time pinpointing the source of the *S. saintpaul* contamination in 2008. Early in the outbreak, the Food and Drug Administration believed the source of *S. saintpaul* to be raw red tomatoes, particularly plum, Roma, and round varieties. But officials never could find a definitive source of contaminated tomatoes. As the list of infected people grew, salsa was considered the common denominator, meaning that not only tomatoes, but cilantro and peppers became suspects as well. It took weeks before FDA investigators traced the source of contamination not to tomatoes, but to jalapeño peppers grown on a farm in Mexico. Later, serrano peppers from another farm in Mexico were implicated as well. Infected tomatoes are still believed to have been the source of the earlier *S. saintpaul* infections, but that hypothesis was never proven. The length of time of the investigation and the lack of definitive sources early on illuminates the vulnerability of this country's fruit and vegetable production and distribution.

Even if the necessary tracking measures are put in place, there is little to prevent contamination from occurring. As such, many people are still uneasy about food grown in distant parts of this country and in foreign countries. Confidence can only be guaranteed when there is complete transparency in the food system. It is not enough for some consumers to know where their food originates and how it got to the supermarket. Rather, these people demand to know—and to see—who is growing their food, where it is growing, and how it is being grown. Many want to talk to the farmers face to face, and even visit their fields and ask direct questions about pesticides and fertilizers. Meeting the people that grow your food builds confidence and trust, and seems to be inherent with locally produced food. While the Associated Press–Ipsos poll was being conducted during the *S. saintpaul* outbreak, a reporter interviewed a grade school teacher in Sacramento, California, about her thoughts on food safety. The teacher acknowledged that she buys most of her fresh produce from the local farmers' markets, and has largely resigned from supermarket produce. Her reasons are simple, "I see the same farmers every single week. You meet the people and you see where the [produce] is coming from."[31] It is this transparency in the food supply that gives people like this Central Valley schoolteacher comfort, and nothing could be more transparent than to have a source of food grown and harvested before your very eyes, as you travel from home to work, school, and places of worship, commerce, and recreation.

The recent outbreaks of pathogen-infected produce have certainly called into question the relative safety of conventional agriculture. But what about urban agriculture? There is a commonly shared perception that small, local farms and community garden plots produce better-tasting, healthier, and safer foods. But are they really safer than their factory-like agribusiness counterparts in remote regions of the world, or at least *as safe*? I posed the question to Marion Nestle, professor of Nutrition, Food Studies, and Public Health at New York University, and author of *Safe Foods: Bacteria, Biotechnology, and Bioterrorism*. Nestle, a proponent of urban agriculture who grows food on her twelfth-floor terrace in New York, acknowledged that the question regarding relative safety of urban- versus rural-grown food is hard to answer definitively. There would need to be testing of the specific produce items, she says; otherwise, we really do not have any way of knowing.[32] But the recent outbreaks of *E. coli* and *Salmonella* provide reasons to believe that there are perhaps inherent risks associated with our centralized system of agriculture that are simply not prevalent with local produce.

A principal reason has to do with distribution. During the *E. coli*-contaminated spinach investigation, health officials determined the bacteria that sickened 200 people in twenty-six states originated from one processor in San Juan Bautista, California. Likewise, the *S. saintpaul* that infected thousands of people across North America in 2008 was traced to a single warehouse in Texas that received shipments from farms in Mexico. Ditto for the *S. typhimurium*-tainted peanut products, where over 700 people across forty-six states fell ill from the products of a single processor in Blakely, Georgia. In each instance, people across the country were sickened by eating produce or produce products originating from one locale.

"The bigger and more global the trade in food," Michael Pollan contends, "the more vulnerable the system is to catastrophe."[33] A decentralized system of many small, local farms and garden plots simply could never have the potential of infecting that many people over so large a geographic area. It was this very pattern of widespread infection that led health officials to conclude that, amid the thousands of people falling ill during the *S. saintpaul* outbreak, produce from local gardens was safe.[34]

Salmonella and *E. coli* are bacteria found in the intestines of animals and humans. So how do they get into our spinach, pepper, peanut, alfalfa, and other produce crops? Usually they come from the feces of animals, meaning that these bacteria can be found in the soil of our "pristine" farm fields (as is the case when fields are fertilized with manure). Or, even more treacherous, bacteria breeds in the water supply used to irrigate the crops. Indeed, irrigation water is a common source of microbial contamination of fresh produce. Large farm fields in the warmer and drier parts of the country (where most of our year-round fresh produce is derived) requires irrigation through large bodies of open water, such as canals and ponds. Open bodies of water present a potential health hazard, as they receive untreated stormwater runoff. When that stormwater finds its way into canals and ponds—after it has been in contact with chicken ranches, feed lots, cow pastures, and other places where concentrations of animal dung can be found—there exists a real risk of contamination. In fact, FDA officials traced the source of the *S. saintpaul* strain that infected serrano peppers to a holding pond used for irrigation.[35] Unlike their rural food-producing counterparts, urban agricultural efforts are at less risk from waterborne pathogens because they are not irrigated by large bodies of open water. Urban gardens are typically irrigated by rainfall and closed sources of potable water, delivered directly to the plants from city waterlines. The chance of contamination from water, therefore, is quite limited.

Of course, crops can also be infected from direct contact with fresh animal dung. This generally results in a more localized contamination, as the bacteria are not spread over an entire field as they are with manure or tainted irrigation water. But the risk is present nonetheless, and some have voiced concern about urban agriculture in public settings, and its proclivity to critters and their bacteria-laden waste.

Animals are attracted to agriculture, certainly, but that attraction is equally strong in rural farm fields as it is on urban plots. In fact, rural fields typically have a greater abundance of livestock and wild critters than our urban settings, and it is much more difficult to secure hundreds of acres of produce from animals than it is smaller garden plots in public spaces.

Admittedly, where there is soil, water, and plants, there will be animals. Unless everything is grown in a secure environment—such as a greenhouse—it is virtually impossible to keep animals away.

Much of the concern regarding animals in urban settings is based largely on misperception. I find it interesting that we often perceive the suburban backyard vegetable garden or the rural farm field as pristine sources of fresh food, free from the harmful waste of animals and other critters. Yet, I recall the animals that are commonly found on rural farm fields: wayward livestock, coyotes, crows, gophers, mice, rabbits, snakes, and lizards. I also recall the animals that I found in my backyard gardens in California and Iowa: skunks, raccoons, deer, rabbits, squirrels, possums, the neighbor's cat (damn that cat!), and all sorts of birds, like cardinals, jays, robins, finches, sparrows, mourning doves, and hummingbirds. The birds, though their feces litter not only my garden but my patio furniture as well, are often welcome creatures to any garden—suburban, urban, or rural. The mammals are a bit more troublesome, for sure, but the fact is that animals will be present wherever food is grown, whether it is the perceived idyllic backyard vegetable garden, the fruit orchard in the neighborhood park, or the small family farm on the outskirts of town.

There may be reason to believe that certain animal waste in cities is safer than in farm fields, however. The CDC notes that reptiles, such as snakes and lizards, "are particularly likely to harbor *Salmonella*."[36] Reptiles are found in great abundance on farm fields, but are less common in urban areas. As such, the risk from *Salmonella* poisoning could be much lower with produce grown in our generally reptile-free cities.

What about human waste? Another concern I occasionally hear regarding planting food in urban spaces is that the homeless will urinate all over the tomatoes and zucchini. Perhaps, although one hopes that homeless people realize that a system of public produce is the community's food supply, feeding not only the homeowners and apartment dwellers in the area, but the homeless themselves. Maybe this is too idealistic. But if one searches for tips on sustainable gardening, and ways to improve the fertility of soil, one finds all sorts of strategies that make a stomach turn. It is well known that urine, high in urea (and thus, nitrogen), is a great fertilizer. Urine is a good source of potassium and phosphorus as well, providing all three macronutrients that plants need. A quick Internet search yields thousands of articles espousing the virtues of human urine and gardening. Even more discomforting for the queasy, some women use their menstrual waste as an organic method of fertilizing their crops.

Human feces, on the other hand, does pose considerable risks if used (or found) in the garden. Though there are a growing number of organizations promoting the benefits of "humanure" (the World Health Organization even published a paper on the topic, citing "the use of excreta and greywater in agriculture is increasingly considered a method combining water and nutrient recycling, increased household food security and improved nutrition for poor households"[37]), it is probably not suitable for smaller agriculture endeavors. The time frame for the breakdown of human manure is too long and the handling requirements too sophisticated for public produce applications.

I realize the benefits of human waste in agriculture may not placate the fastidious, since we have become a society accustomed to produce with a shiny wax coating, packaged on polystyrene trays and shrink-wrapped in cellophane. The bottom line is that all produce, whether purchased from the supermarket or the farmers' market, or grown in our backyard or a downtown parking lot, has undoubtedly come into contact with animals and insects, microbes and bacteria, and should therefore be thoroughly washed before consumption. And if there are particular public spaces with known problems of animal infestations or human encampments, then perhaps the best strategy is to seek another public plot.

Our industrial-scale, centralized system of food production is more susceptible not only to accidental contaminations from microbes, but to malicious terrorist tampering as well. Bioterrorism is a growing concern in this country, and for good reason. According to Marion Nestle, the demands placed on the Food and Drug Administration (which is tasked with monitoring the safety of the nation's fruit and vegetable supply and production, including imports), are unreasonable. Nestle reports, "About 700 FDA inspectors must oversee 30,000 food manufacturers and processors, 20,000 warehouses, 785,000 commercial and institutional food establishments, 128,000 grocery and convenience stores, and 1.5 million vending operations. The agency must also deal with food imports, which comprised 40% of the country's supply of fresh fruits and vegetables and 68% of the seafood in 2000."[38]

Because of the monumental burden placed on this severely understaffed government body, Nestle concludes that "it is not surprising that the FDA conducted only 5,000 inspections annually, visited less than 2% of the places under its jurisdiction, and inspected less than 1% of imported foods prior to 2001 when threats of bioterrorism forced improvements."[39]

The improvements Nestle alluded to have done little to boost confidence over our nation's food supply with regard to bioterrorism. During a press conference in 2004, after improvements to the FDA's funding and staffing were in place, Tommy Thompson, then secretary of Health and Human Services, offered a most chilling admission. Thompson told his audience, "I, for the life of me, cannot understand why the terrorists have not attacked our food supply, because it is so easy to do."[40] Michael Pollan agrees. "When a single factory is grinding 20 million hamburger patties in a week or washing 25 million servings of salad, a single terrorist armed with a canister of toxins can, at a stroke, poison millions." Pollan argues that "the best way to protect our food system against such threats is obvious: decentralize it."[41]

Another concern over the relative safety of conventional agriculture has to do with policing the use of the myriad—and potentially harmful—agrichemicals. It is difficult to say what happens on those large agricultural fields in remote parts of the country with regard to the application of chemical fertilizers, pesticides, herbicides, or other contaminants. And when our food is grown in other countries, all bets are off (recall China's melamine-contaminated milk scandal in 2008).

The use of agrichemicals in conventional agriculture is for one purpose only: to increase profit by maximizing yields of saleable produce. As such, agrichemicals are often liberally sprayed on farm fields, and sometimes, on farmworkers. One instance involving Ag-Mart (a prominent grower of tomatoes in North Carolina and Florida) and one of its field workers presents some of the grotesque effects that result from a person's direct exposure to agrichemicals.

Carlos Herrera Candelario was born without arms or legs, and with abnormalities to his lungs and spine—the result of, according to his mother, repeated exposure to pesticides while she was pregnant. Carlos's mother claimed she and other field workers were often doused with pesticides while they harvested tomatoes. Ag-Mart denies any wrongdoing, claiming the charges against the company are "a misreading of its records."[42] But in a three-month period between December 2004 and February 2005, three deformed children, Carlos included, were born to Ag-Mart field workers. Shortly afterward, Ag-Mart terminated its use of five pesticides that are known to cause birth defects. Without admitting guilt, Ag-Mart settled with Carlos's parents, agreeing to pay for his lifelong care.

Monetary profits are not generally the desired goal with urban public gardens, so maximum yields may be neither necessary nor desired. And people today generally desire organically grown produce. The problem is they cannot afford to buy organic, so they choose the cheaper, chemically grown produce. But with a system of public produce, where it is not financial gain that is sought, but community health, there is less reason to use chemical fertilizers, pesticides, and herbicides in the management of our urban food systems.

While urban soils may be free (or freer) of agrichemicals, there is one contaminant that concerns many with regard to growing food in cities: lead.

Lead is often found in the grounds of our older city neighborhoods and former industrial areas. A common misperception, however, is that the presence of lead in soil automatically disqualifies any agricultural endeavor. Another misperception is that all urban soils are contaminated. There are generally just two sources for lead contamination in urban soils: lead-based paint, where peeling paint from buildings has fallen and mixed with the soil, and emissions from automobiles that ran on leaded gasoline. As such, the areas in the city where lead contamination may be likely are on the sites of old paint factories, gas stations, and vacant lots where old buildings have been razed; near foundations of old buildings that may have been painted with lead-based paint; and within a couple feet of busy streets. While lead has typically been absent in paint and gasoline for quite some time, it moves little in the soil, creating a persistent concern for contamination.

According to a report by Carl Rosen, a soil scientist with the University of Minnesota Extension, "The most serious source of exposure to soil lead is through direct ingestion (eating) of contaminated soil or dust. In general, plants do not absorb or accumulate lead." Rosen goes on to note that "since plants do not take up large quantities of soil lead, the lead levels in soil considered safe for plants will be much higher than soil lead levels where eating of soil is a concern (pica). Generally, it has been considered safe to use garden produce grown in soils with total lead levels less than 300 ppm."

At these levels and lower, Rosen reports, "Studies have shown that lead does not readily accumulate in the fruiting parts of vegetable and fruit crops (e.g., corn, beans, squash, tomatoes, strawberries, apples)." Rosen states that leafy vegetables are more likely to absorb lead from the soil, but that there is "more concern about lead contamination from external lead on unwashed produce than from actual uptake by the plant itself."[43] The suggested remedy for external lead contamination? Wash your produce.

A simple site test is advised if the presence of lead in the soil is suspected. If lead is found, it may not be necessary to seek another plot to garden. As Rosen advises, contaminations of less than 300 parts per million are generally safe to garden without any soil remediation. If levels are higher, or if municipal officials want added peace of mind, there are numerous remedies to ensure safe, contaminant-free produce.

The most common is to create raised beds on top of the existing soil. Because lead moves very little in the soil, the risk of contaminating the upper soil is generally nil. Because lead tends to stay put, it is generally concentrated in the top three to four inches of existing soil. Another strategy is to excavate to this depth, replacing the contaminated soil with fresh, clean topsoil, which virtually guarantees contamination-free produce. A third strategy is to keep the soil pH neutral (i.e., 7.0), the level where the vast majority of plants thrive anyway. This can be done with common soil amendments. Soils with a pH of 6.5 or higher immobilize lead, rendering it unavailable to plants.

Other urban soil contaminants, such as paints, solvents, oil, gas, and other chemicals, are typically found in the same areas where lead can be common: gas stations, paint factories, and other former industrial sites. Municipal officials often desire to return these brownfields to green, and the remediation strategies for lead can be as successful as with other contaminants. Public space sites, however—such as parks, plazas, and town squares that were never previously developed, or subjected to chemical spills—are likely

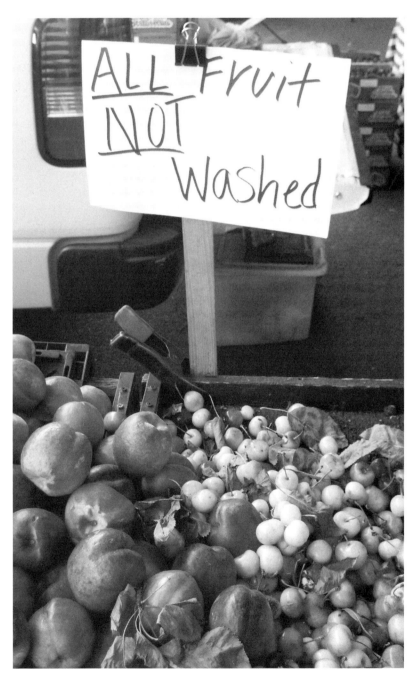

Even farmers' market produce needs to be washed, as this vendor reminds us.

clean, requiring little remediation, if any. Still, a common soil test is recommended for any agriculture endeavor, rural or urban. If contaminants are found, and remediation proves too costly, sage advice is to simply find another site. The beauty of public-space cultivation is that there are many suitable—and clean—sites throughout the city.

There will always be risks associated with growing and consuming food. Some concerns are valid, though most are based on naïveté. Nevertheless, these perceptions may prove to be formidable obstacles to implementing a public produce program in many communities. The truth is that farms today have few regulations in place to ensure absolute safety of fruits and vegetables, and there is perhaps greater potential for municipal government and its citizenry to work together to ensure a healthier and safer food system.

If cities and their citizenry are to live on and realize enduring vigor and vitality, local systems of food production will have to be unearthed. As Michael Pollan notes, "The American people are paying more attention to food today than they have in decades, worrying not only about its price but about its safety, its provenance and its healthfulness. There is a gathering sense among the public that the industrial-food system is broken."[44] Pollan argues that until we address the flawed food system that feeds Americans, food security—and hence, national security—is compromised. James Howard Kunstler's claims are perhaps more dire. His apocalyptic forecast was easy to dismiss as a doomsday rant when *The Long Emergency* was published in 2005. But in the short time since, Kunstler's predictions are proving not only plausible, but imminent. For Kunstler, local food production in the twenty-first century is a simple issue of community existence: Those who produce their own food will continue to exist; those who cannot, will wither and die.

Though Pollan's and Kunstler's arguments tend toward hyperbole, their underlying message is grounded and lucid. The current agriculture system in America is proving vulnerable, and we need strategies to create a more secure food supply, for the health of our environment, our economy, and our people. Is large-scale agribusiness going away? Probably not. Is it reasonable for Americans to completely return to an agrarian lifestyle in and immediately near our cities? Doubtful. Is it possible to add fresh-produce choices and agricultural efforts in our urban settings, exploiting the food-producing potential of our current network of underutilized public spaces? Indubitably.

Chapter 2

The Cost of Healthy Calories

COLIN BEAVAN, KNOWN BY MANY AS NO IMPACT MAN, set out on a year-long journey to find homeostasis, an equilibrium between his consumerist way of life and environmentalist ideals. His goal was deceptively modest: to sustain a simple life in New York City without making any net impact on the environment. To Beavan, that meant "no trash, no carbon emissions, no toxins in the water, no elevators, no subway, no products in packaging, no plastics, no air conditioning, no TV, no toilets. . . ."[1] And it also meant a very different way of eating. Beavan needed to eschew fast and processed foods, and only consume locally raised, organically grown foods to be honest to the No Impact Man project. At the end of his experiment, Beavan realized that "eating local is a no-brainer if you live in a rich neighborhood with the cool, local-food farmers' market nearby." Beavan has received criticism that his experiment was bourgeois, and he now understands why. "Not consuming resources is no problem if a life of purchasing power has provided you with most of what you need," he admits. It is quite perplexing that to live a simple lifestyle in America is beyond the financial means of many. It is easy to say that we all should buy more organic, locally grown produce. It is quite another to be able to do so. And as Beavan has discovered, "Nutritious, local food should not just be available to the wealthy while the poor are left with McDonalds and KFC."[2]

Beavan's discovery of the conundrum between local, organically grown food and its high cost brings us to another important consideration in food security: public health. We've all seen the emaciated bodies of starving people living in countries crippled by food insecurity. It is oxymoronic that obesity is the result of food insecurity here in America. It is not the inaccessibility of food calories in this country that is problematic. Rather, it is the abundance of cheap calories derived from processed and fast food vis-à-vis the inaccessibility of fresh, wholesome, nutrient-dense foods at an affordable price that is responsible for the poor health of this nation's citizens.

We have found, through subsidizing grain crops and economies of scale, how to produce fast and processed foods in much larger quantities and at cheaper prices than we can produce fresh fruits and vegetables. The bulk of corn produced in this country, for example, does not go to feed people directly. Rather, it is used primarily for silage to feed anything from cows (that produce meat, cheese, and milk), to chickens (meat and eggs) to hogs, and even to fish raised in fish farms. Corn is also processed into corn oil and high-fructose corn syrup, which has found its way into practically all of our baked goods, cereals, soft drinks, juice drinks, and other processed foods. In short, we have become a nation of corn.[3]

Corn—or more specifically, corn-derived food products—has now become the staple in the American diet. But cheeseburgers, soda pop, and snack foods have traditionally been regarded as luxury items, not staples; at least, they are not typically staples in those countries eating a traditional, non-Western diet. And certainly high-fructose corn syrup should be a luxury item or treat, as it is simply a sweetener. But through our subsidized and industrialized system of agriculture, we are able to produce these highly processed luxury items so that they compete in price with fresh fruits and vegetables, nuts, seeds, pulses, legumes, and other grains—the types of food that should be staples in our diet.

Michael Pollan argues that "the surest way to escape the Western diet is simply to depart the realms it rules: the supermarket, the convenience store, and the fast-food outlet."[4] Instead, Pollan recommends eating more food from farmers' markets and community-supported agriculture groups. Easier said than done for some people. Consider this: you can purchase a large, fresh, organic peach at the farmers' market for one dollar, or a double cheeseburger from the McDonald's Dollar Menu. The peach has 73 calories and less than one gram of fat. The double cheeseburger has 440 calories, and twenty-three grams of fat.[5] Which do you choose if you are hungry, impoverished, and living in a low-income neighborhood, and only have a dollar in your pocket? It is really a trick question, as it is almost impossible to find fresh produce in economically depressed neighborhoods anyway. Fast food, on the other hand, is ubiquitous. It is a harsh reality in a capitalist economy that supermarkets, farmers' markets, and grocery stores simply do not locate in impoverished neighborhoods, leaving residents with a dearth of food options.

Community food activist Mark Winne calls these impoverished areas food deserts—"places with too few choices of healthy and affordable food, and [that] are oversaturated with unhealthy food outlets such as fast food joints." Winne explains that "while the failure of supermarkets to adequately serve lower-income communities represents a failure of the marketplace, the marketplace is functioning rationally (as economists would say) by going to where the money is." The consequential health outlook for people living in these food deserts is quite predictable. Residents of these areas,

Winne notes, "tend to be poorer and have fewer healthy food options, which in turn contributes to their high overweight/obesity rates and diet-related illnesses such as diabetes."[6]

Huntington, West Virginia, is one such food desert—perhaps the most barren in the nation. Once a proud and fairly prosperous coal-mining town, Huntington now carries the shameful moniker of the unhealthiest city in America, according to statistics from the Centers for Disease Control and Prevention (CDC). Almost 50 percent of adults in the Huntington metro region are obese. And that is just the beginning of the city's health problems. Huntington leads the nation in heart disease, diabetes, and tooth decay. Nearly half of all elderly adults in Huntington have lost all of their natural teeth—an astounding statistic that no other city in the country can come close to. A nurse at St. Mary's Regional Heart Institute in Huntington notes that many patients are suffering from heart attacks in their thirties. At an age that is considered the prime of life in other parts of the country, people in Huntington are getting open-heart surgeries. Hot dog eateries abound in Huntington. The city has more pizza places than the entire state of West Virginia has health clubs and gyms. "Fast food has become the staple," noted a manager within the state health department, "with many residents convinced they can't afford to buy healthier foods." A retired policeman blamed the economy, stating it needed to pick up "so people can afford to get healthy." The city's mayor underwent stomach surgery to help him lose weight, yet he has no desire to curb the fast-food eateries that proliferate in Huntington. "We want as much business as we can have here," notes the mayor. "As many restaurants as you have, it kind of enhances the livability. Maybe not the health."[7]

On the other side of the country, municipal attitudes toward fast-food restaurants are considerably different. In the summer of 2008, the Los Angeles city council garnered national attention when it unanimously approved a one-year moratorium on fast-food restaurants within a particularly food-bleak section of their city. South Los Angeles (formerly South Central, if you recall) is one of the more expansive food deserts in America, occupying thirty-two square miles and inhabited by half a million people. Like Huntington, the swelling of fast-food eateries in South L.A. is reflected in the community's expanding waistlines. This urban area has the highest concentration of fast-food eateries and the lowest number of grocery stores in the city. Thirty percent of South Los Angeles residents are obese, far greater than the 19 percent for the metropolitan region and 14 percent for the affluent area of Westside.[8] Residents of South Los Angeles also have the highest incidence of diabetes in Los Angeles County (remember Ron Finley's observation? "Dialysis centers are popping up like Starbucks!"). To the city council, the need to suspend fast-food eateries is obvious. The health of their citizens is at stake, and the moratorium buys the municipality time to attract healthier food outlets.

As you might have expected, restaurant associations and representatives of fast-food chains were dismayed, claiming the moratorium on fast food is misguided, and does not guarantee the emergence of healthier food options. And even if those healthier food options emerge, will they be affordable to the people of South Los Angeles?

According to Kelly Brownell, director of the Rudd Center for Food Policy and Obesity at Yale University, people will change their diet when different foods are offered, but cost becomes an important factor in poor communities. Curtis English, a South Los Angeles resident who was interviewed by a reporter covering the moratorium, put the food problem in proper perspective. English recognizes that fast food is loaded with calories and cholesterol. But since he is unemployed and does not own a car, he is most concerned with how far he can stretch his food dollar within his neighborhood. English recalled that he ate at a McDonald's within a few blocks of his home twice the day before the city council passed the moratorium. For a mere $2.39, English had a sausage burrito for breakfast and a double cheeseburger for lunch. While Brownell notes that "diets improve when healthy food establishments enter these neighborhoods,"[9] the real cost consideration is just how many healthful calories can one buy for $2.39?

A moratorium on fast-food establishments is a good start, but only solves one part of a more complex problem. As long as America is a capitalist nation, it is foolhardy to assume that supermarkets, farmers' markets, and restaurants with fresh, wholesome offerings will flock to distressed communities. The real solution boils down to accessibility *and* affordability. One strategy, and perhaps an effective one, is for the municipality to cultivate a policy that exploits the food-growing and distribution potential of public spaces within these communities, to ensure that fresh, wholesome food is, at the very least, as prevalent as fast food, and just as cheap (or preferably, cheaper).

Though the fast-food moratorium was controversial, the efforts of the City of Los Angeles should be lauded, as they illuminate the need for municipal planners and local government to tackle food insecurity in their communities head on. Many communities across the nation have placed restrictions on fast-food restaurants, but they usually cite architectural design or preservation of historical character as their reason. Los Angeles may be the only municipality in recent history to cite public health as the reason for its restriction. Though many object to having government interfere with private industry, the municipality's actions are really just an example of sound urban planning. A moratorium on fast-food businesses is no different from prohibiting a liquor store or an adult book store from locating near schools, for example, or requiring that manufacturing and heavy industry be segregated from housing. As David Zinczenko, editor in chief of *Men's Health* magazine and the author of several diet books, reasons, "What we're beginning to see is almost the monopolization of our dietary intake by a handful of corporations. Add to that the financial reality of feeding ourselves today, where a single grapefruit from a corner fruit stand costs two or more times as much as a few Chicken McNuggets, and I think you can begin to put together a case for governmental intervention."[10] Los Angeles's moratorium on fast food demonstrates that municipality's belief that providing access to healthier food options falls well within the regimen of city planning and local public policy. At the very least, the council's actions open a dialogue about the specific roles city government can play to protect the community's health and welfare. Critics will continue to argue that the moratorium limits food choices, though the City of Los Angeles argues the contrary. The choice between fast food or no food is no choice at all. Los Angeles will, I predict, set a new trend in the planning and development of our cities, using food and public health as an organizer of city reform.

It cannot be overstated: people living in dire conditions in this country need access to affordable, fresh, wholesome food in order to improve their health. Without regular access to cheap-yet-nutrient-dense foods, our nation's waistline will continue to expand, and our health decline.

The CDC reports that obesity rates across the American population have risen dramatically over the past three decades (a trend that coincides with the increase in availability of processed and fast foods). In 1990, for example, not a single state in this country reported a prevalence of obesity that was greater than 15 percent of its adult population. By 2010, not a single state could make that claim.[11] Every state in the nation reported a prevalence of obesity that was greater than 20 percent of its adult population by 2010. Today, more than 35 percent of adults aged twenty years and older are obese in the United States. What is more alarming is the increase of obese children, from the very young to young adults. Data collected from two National Health and Nutrition Examination Surveys (1976–1980 and 2003–2006) illustrate this disconcerting trend. For children two to five years old, the prevalence of obesity "increased from 5.0% to 12.4%; for those aged 6–11 years, prevalence increased from 6.5% to 17.0%; and for those aged 12–19 years, prevalence increased from 5.0% to 17.6%."[12]

Obesity is also costly. In 2008, the CDC estimated that the medical costs for people who are obese were $1,429 higher than those who are a normal weight.[13] That is because obesity increases the risk of contracting type 2 diabetes, heart disease, stroke, and certain types of cancer—interminable ailments with expensive treatments. When you factor in the sheer numbers of the obese in this country, the medical bills are staggering. Obesity costs Americans 147 *billion* dollars each year.[14]

The CDC has labeled American society "obesogenic," a condition resulting from "environments that promote increased food intake, nonhealthful foods, and physical inactivity."[15] Because we have created a culture inclined toward a sedentary, overindulgent lifestyle, the CDC notes that the only way we can halt obesity is through changes in policy and our environment. The CDC's Division of Nutrition, Physical Activity and Obesity outlines six strategies to curb obesity, four of which focus on food. In addition to increasing physical activity and decreasing television viewing, the CDC recommends that Americans decrease the consumption of sugar-sweetened beverages; decrease the consumption of high-energy-dense foods; increase breast-feeding initiation and duration for newborns; and increase consumption of fruits and vegetables. Only 27 percent of adults in America are eating the recommended three servings of vegetables per day, and only 33 percent are meeting their daily recommendation of two servings of fruit.[16]

The link between fresh produce and public health is so strong that even health care organizations are devising strategies to increase accessibility to fresh fruits and vegetables. Kaiser Permanente, one of the largest healthcare organizations in the country, has recently instituted farmers' markets on the hospital grounds of many of their facilities. Preston Maring, a Kaiser physician, came up with the idea for a farmers' market after he noticed the success of the jewelry and handbag vendors hawking their wares in the lobby of the Oakland hospital where he practices. A firm believer of the connection between food, diet, and health, Maring thought a modest produce stand or farmers' market could be an amenity for patients and staff as well, perhaps even functioning as a form of preventative medicine. In 2003, the first Kaiser Permanente farmers' market opened outside the lobby of the Oakland hospital. Two years later, two dozen more opened in five states. By 2012, over fifty farmers' markets operated in the parking lots of Kaiser Permanente, from Georgia to Hawaii. What began as an idea by a pioneering physician in Oakland, California, became a staple for Kaiser Permanente across the country, and a manifestation of Maring's belief that "nothing is more important to people's health than what they eat every day."[17]

A bad diet affects not only physical health, but mental ability as well. According to a study published in the April 2008 edition of *Journal of School Health*, students with an increased intake of fruits and vegetables fared better on standardized literacy assessments than children on diets high in junk food.[18] For this reason, and others regarding physical health, it is imperative that children have access to a plentiful variety of fresh fruit and vegetables at home, at school, and on their way to and from these places.

Children are impressionable, and they tend to crave what they see around them. They are especially susceptible to the marketing blitzes of the big processed- and fast-food companies. If children see nothing but ads promoting fast-food meals, they will want fast-food meals. A common ploy in supermarket chains is to place the sugary cereals, cookies, and other junk foods at eye level of children. This strategy might be tolerable if the marketing blitz were balanced with equally eye-popping graphics of fictional characters and personified animals touting healthy foods. Such is not the case. According to an article in the *New York Times*, "almost three-fourths of the advertising aimed at children is for candy, snacks, sugary cereals or fast food."[19] Sweden bans all advertising aimed at children under twelve years old. Many other European countries restrict television ads during children's programming. But in the United States, marketing to "kid kustomers" is big business, as

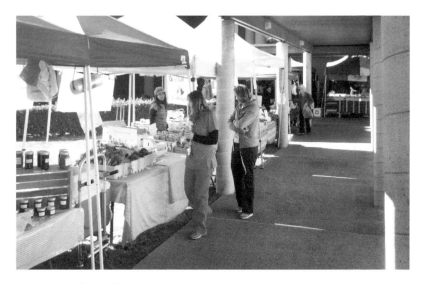

Hospital staff shop for fresh, locally grown produce at this farmers' market at Kaiser Permanente (California).

companies hope to snare brand loyalty at a young age, ensuring a customer for life.[20]

It is doubtful that Americans will pass legislation banning advertising to our kids anytime soon. Until then, healthy foods need to be just as visible and accessible as junk foods, preferably more so. Infusing our public spaces with fresh produce can help mitigate the marketing inundation of processed and fast foods, and actually teach children about the cycles of life, whole foods, and where those whole foods come from. If children really do crave what they see most often, ensuring the ubiquity of fresh produce is a strategy worthy of exploration.

Poor diet is not the only variable in obesity. Our sedentary lifestyle works to expand our waistline as well, and doctors routinely remind us that proper diet and exercise are the keys to healthful living. It is time to think how our public spaces could improve public health by providing places for exercise and access to healthy food.

For example, the CDC states that one effective measure for combating obesity is to seek opportunities for physical activity within the community, such as hiking and biking along trails in parks and sidewalks along city streets. Not only could these public spaces provide opportunities for physical activity, but with the planting of fruits and vegetables, public space can increase access to the fresh produce that is necessary in (and largely missing from) American diets.

Such an example is already in place in Davenport, Iowa. Genesis Health System, a locally owned and operated health care facility for the Quad Cities, recently added a modern outdoor exercise station within the city's Duck Creek Parkway. In addition to the greenbelt's existing bicycle paths, playgrounds, and various sports fields and courts, the new fitness station offers another choice in physical activity. Genesis officials could not have erected their new exercise station in a more propitious location, near the shade of two very large apple trees. These remnants of what was likely a modest orchard provide the only clues to what existed here before the municipality purchased the farmstead and turned it into parkland. But those vestiges of local food production are strong. As the creek trickles by and cyclists pedal along its meandering path, people stair-step, push up, flex, and stretch, while red orbs of ripe fruit hang tantalizingly overhead. This active scene in such a serene setting sparks the desire for a healthier, more environmentally enriching lifestyle. Though there is a certain pastoral character to this particular park, the experience is uniquely urban. It is these experiences, rare today, that offer promise of a more bountiful, healthful, food-secure city.

Chapter 3

Public Space, Public Officials, Public Policy

Nathan Murray is not your typical farmer. Sure, he has the stocky build of a man who works the land. But he is a white-collar green thumber who tends his crops in Dockers, loafers, and a Van Heusen. Murray's smart casual attire—perhaps a bit spiffy for growing vegetables—is actually mandatory. He is a representative of City Hall, after all.

"Pansies have their place, but I prefer looking at tomatoes," Murray admits. Murray—a city planner for the City of Provo, Utah—is referring to the view out his cubicle window. The raised brick planters dotting the plaza on the south side of City Hall used to be planted with the usual flashy suspects: pansies, petunias, and marigolds. But those showy flowers have long been replaced by equally showy fruits, like tomatoes, peppers, and eggplant. And Murray is the reason for the change in the landscape's visage.

Murray's transformation of City Hall's landscape was sparked by an all-too-familiar story. During the economic freefall that tipped in 2008, municipalities across the nation tightened their belts. In an effort to cut costs, "minimum maintenance" became the mantra bellowed from the halls of every municipal building in America. Budgets for landscaping the city's public spaces and buildings were slashed. Flowers were luxuries municipalities couldn't afford. Even if they could, such displays were certainly not evocative of fiscally prudent budget managers.

But Murray didn't want to look out his cubicle window and see empty dirt. Besides, this was City Hall, a prestigious civic building that should convey a friendly and inviting message to the public, not an austere one.

Murray had just finished reading a book on guerilla gardening, and that sprouted an idea. He would commandeer those empty planters and fill them with vegetables. His goals were quite simple: to provide a bit of greenery to soften the stark plaza around City Hall, and to show folks just how much food can be produced from a little bit of dirt.

He began by germinating vegetable seeds in a makeshift green-house—in this case his cubicle. With the office thermostat set to 72 degrees and the flood of light from the overhead fluorescent tubes, Murray's cubicle proved an ideal environment to sprout to-matoes, peppers, melons, squash, eggplant, beans, and all sorts of heat-loving plants . . . even in the dead of winter. Once the danger of frost had passed, Murray and a couple coworkers transplanted their City Hall seedlings outside. They may not have realized it at the time, but their simple act of planting food in public space would prove wildly popular.

Murray and his colleagues started the City Hall veggie patch in spring of 2009, and they've never looked back. The vegetables immediately garnered the admiration of coworkers, the mayor (who lauded the garden in his blog[1]), the public, and news crews throughout Provo. Murray and his gardening crew have been

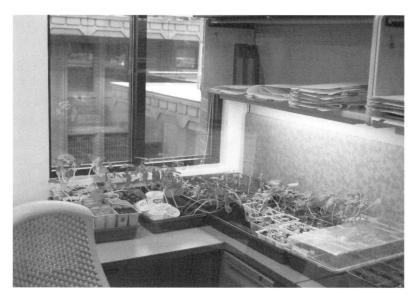

A temperature-controlled office cubicle with fluorescent lights proves to be an excellent environment for germinating vegetable seeds in the dead of winter. (Courtesy of Nathan Murray, City of Provo)

featured in numerous blogs, newspapers, and television news segments. It seems growing food in public space for the benefit of the public has great appeal to the folks of Provo.

During that first year, Murray harvested about 300 pounds of produce, which was donated to the local food bank. In 2010, Murray *doubled* the harvest. By 2012, Murray and his coworkers were able to coax 1,200 pounds of vegetables from those same planters, whose surface area, when aggregated, totals a scant 250 square feet of dirt. Murray's thumb became forest green in just a few short years. Not only that, but he realized his goal: you *can* grow an awful lot of food in a small amount of space.

Since the garden had been so successful the first few years, in 2013 Murray decided to relocate to a vacant lot three blocks away. The parcel gave him far more real estate to work with, and planting a garden could do a lot to improve the public image of the neglected site. But Murray learned an invaluable lesson that year: site selection for public produce is paramount for its success.

"People didn't see the garden has having as much significance," noted Murray. "It wasn't as special, having vegetables growing on a vacant lot versus City Hall."[2] Indeed, vacant lot gardening, though a fantastic endeavor for land that otherwise lies fallow, doesn't make us do a double take, pause, and think the way that seeing growing food in true civic space does. There is tremendous power in the example. Like First Lady Michelle Obama's garden on the South Lawn at the White House, growing vegetables at City Hall sends a symbolic message about food and our food culture. "Gosh, if City Hall is advocating fresh, locally grown tomatoes, zucchini, and cucumbers, maybe I should think twice about ordering that double cheeseburger for lunch. And maybe I should start gardening, too."

Murray also noticed that the vacant lot garden was more difficult to maintain than the City Hall planters. Because the garden wasn't deemed as special, it was tougher for Murray to motivate coworkers to help tend crops. Not only that, but gardening is much more convenient when it is right outside your door. Pulling the occasional weed as you return to the office from lunch, or turning on the hose during your morning break are tasks that become almost effortless, simply because you are passing by the garden multiple times each day. The new garden was a short walk from City Hall. But it doesn't matter. As soon as you have to go out of your way to weed, water, or even harvest ripe produce, gardening becomes a chore.

For 2014, Murray admitted the garden needs to return to City Hall; not only for the prestige, but for ease of maintenance. And speaking of maintenance, it should be noted that Murray and his colleagues tend the crops on their own time, usually before or after work, and sometimes on their lunch break. This is quite generous of the city planners in Provo, but I asked Murray, "Even with the gardens right outside your door, doesn't the maintenance still consume a lot of your free time?"

"I'm surprised how much can be done with just a little bit of effort," Murray told me. "It doesn't take much to turn over a section of dirt, throw in some seeds, and remember to water. If you can weed every now and again, all the better, and the yield is rather remarkable."[3]

What Murray has learned is that a lot of food and community good can be nurtured with just a little time and a modest patch of soil. As a public official, Murray is one of the many stewards of public space in his city, and his many years of growing food in those civic planters has changed Murray's attitude about urban space. "The space we planted was grossly underutilized, as are a lot of city-owned spaces," Murray admitted. "It was good to put it to a higher and better use."

Now, whenever he passes by some underutilized piece of land, like an empty corner in a park or a forgotten parking strip along the street, Murray says, "I just want to throw some strawberries in there."[4]

When folks hear "urban agriculture," what often comes to mind are community gardens on vacant parcels in distressed neighborhoods, similar to what Murray planted in 2013. But urban agriculture is much more diverse. Former San Francisco mayor Gavin Newsom once said, "Urban agriculture is about far more than growing vegetables on an empty lot. It's about revitalizing and transforming unused public spaces, connecting city residents with their neighborhoods in a new way and promoting healthier eating and living for everyone."[5]

Newsom's statement was in reference to a pioneering food policy he was championing in 2009. At the time, Newsom was urging municipalities to lead the fight against food insecurity. The mayor laid out a comprehensive agriculture plan for the city, to bolster access to fresh fruits and vegetables and reshape how San Franciscans think about food.

Newsom kicked off his agricultural plan with an Executive Directive, which declares, "Access to safe, nutritious, and culturally acceptable food is a basic human right and is essential to both human health and ecological sustainability. The City and County of San Francisco recognizes that hunger, food insecurity, and poor nutrition are pressing health issues that require immediate action." The Directive then states, "Food production and horticulture education will be encouraged within the City and, to the extent feasible, on City owned land." The Directive concludes with a set of action steps, the first one stating, "All [City] departments having jurisdiction over property will conduct an audit of their land suitable for or actively used for food producing gardens or other agricultural purposes."[6] This meant the Department of Public Works would look at the potential to grow food on land they oversee, namely streets. Recreation and Parks would look at city parks; the Planning Department would look at vacant parcels they have acquired; the Public Library would analyze the grounds around their buildings to grow food; and so on.

Newsom's food policy might be ahead of its time, but only slightly. The declining health of our nation is directly linked to our poor diet and, as Newsom noted, requires immediate action. Every municipality aims to improve the quality of life for its citizens, and one of the surest, most effective strategies to achieve such an aim is to adopt an urban agriculture policy similar to the one that Newsom has outlined for San Francisco.

Newsom's Directive illustrates the variety of public spaces worthy of agricultural exploration. Though the community garden on the vacant lot will likely continue to epitomize urban agriculture, as the practice evolves, it will become clear that the diversity of public space within cities presents a diversity of food-growing opportunities.

I should clarify that, by "public space," I am referring to those places that are freely accessible to the public, whether they are truly public or merely perceived to be. True public spaces include those properties owned and maintained by the municipality, such as streets and sidewalks, parks, squares and plazas, parking lots, and municipal buildings (libraries, city halls, and police and fire stations, for example, and the landscaped grounds that surround them). Civic institutions not owned by the municipality, but by other government or public agencies, may also be public, such as courthouses, universities, and grade schools. Then there are those spaces that are privately owned, but where permission to pass is explicitly stated or implied. Hospitals, business parks, churches, corporate plazas, retail and commercial parking lots are examples of privately owned spaces where the public freely enters, and is often encouraged to do so. Even floodplains and transportation and utility easements, where structures are not allowed to be built, can be great opportunities for food production. In essence, any space where the public can enter throughout the day without being charged an admission fee (even if that space is privately owned and maintained), and is suitable for growing food, is worthy of inclusion in a network of public produce.

I am not advocating the removal of fountains, benches, paving, sculpture, playground equipment, picnic tables, and other public-space amenities that attract people for the sake of urban agriculture. Quite the contrary. I am interested in ways of attracting *more* people, by providing additional reasons for folks to frequent public space: namely, wholesome sustenance, food education, and a sense of self-sufficiency.

In the design of public spaces, there are many variables that, when properly identified and accommodated for, work together to create vivacity. Food is often one of those variables. This was something the late preeminent people-watcher William H. Whyte recognized over thirty years ago. In his seminal book *The Social Life of Small Urban Spaces*, Whyte proffered, "If you want to seed a place with activity, put out food." That's because, he writes, "Food attracts people who attract more people." Whyte was so convinced of the positive impacts food has on the attractiveness of public space that he reiterated, just a couple paragraphs later, "Food, to repeat, draws people, and they draw more people."[7]

What Whyte was speaking about in particular was food prepared and sold from vendors, which helps make the many street corners and plazas in Manhattan so attractive to the passerby. But we are starting to witness an utter fascination with the *growing* of food as well. Gardens and orchards can be community gathering places, and food—even fresh produce in its natural habitat—can improve the attractiveness of public space, and its ability to create a sense of conviviality.

It matters little if the space is truly public or only semipublic—municipal government is going to have to play a leading role in shaping food policy, as Mayor Newsom argued. Programs, policies, funding strategies, and maintenance regimens of any urban agriculture endeavor will be difficult to implement and sustain if the largest landowner in the city is indifferent. If public officials want a healthier, more prosperous citizenry, and believe that access to fresh, locally sourced, wholesome, and affordable food is good for both the individual citizen and the community at large, then public officials can no longer remain idle. In the face of rising food insecurity and declining public health stemming from a poor diet, public officials need to provide better food choices in their community.

Which is exactly what the City of Calgary is doing.

The same year Mayor Newsom unveiled his municipal agriculture plan for San Francisco, the City of Calgary broke ground on the Community Orchard Research Project, a five-year pilot program testing public fruit trees and their ability to thrive in urban settings and a harsh climate. "We have a grassland landscape, not a woodland landscape," noted Jill Spence, lead urban forester with the City of Calgary, as she outlined the challenges of growing fruit trees in her region. "Plus, it gets very cold here, then you have Chinooks which can wreak havoc on the budding cycle of fruit trees."

Such natural constraints would be enough for most municipal governments to forego any attempt to plant fruit trees for the community. Heck, even in cities with mild climates, most public officials wouldn't entertain an opportunity to plant produce in public settings. But the City of Calgary sees food differently. "Food in Calgary is a priority," Spence said. "It improves our urban forest, engages our community, and improves our image. For Calgarians, this is important."[8]

The idea for the orchards didn't come from Spence, or the City of Calgary. Rather, it came from the community. Though you might expect most bureaucrats to rattle off a litany of reasons why fruit trees shouldn't be planted in public spaces, the City of Calgary listened to its citizens. Spence then engaged the experts at the University of Saskatchewan to determine which fruit trees and shrubs might do best in Calgary's challenging environment. Apples, pears, apricots, honeyberries, hazelnuts, gooseberries, and cherries were some of the fruits recommended by the university.

So Spence and her crew set to work planting orchards in four public parks. And they didn't start timidly. For the Sunnyside Community Orchard, thirty apple, three pear, thirty cherry, five apricot, seventy-eight honeyberry, fifty-five strawberry, seventeen gooseberry, and six hazelnut trees and shrubs were planted. We're not talking a few fruit trees to appease a citizen request, but a veritable fruit farm that rivals any small commercial orchard.

In fact, it was precisely the commercial orchard that the City of Calgary modeled their pilot project after. "We are taking a different approach from a hobby garden," says Russell Friesen, an urban forester who works with Spence. "We are trying to take a more economic approach and something closer to commercial orchards, using commercial varieties."

Friesen noted that the apple varieties used for the city's orchard project use dwarf root stock, meaning the trees will only get to be six or seven feet tall. "They are easy picking, and these dwarf trees invest more energy in the fruit than they do in the wood," says Friesen. "They're not particularly esthetically pleasing: they look weird. But for the purposes of a community orchard, the best practice is to grow on these dwarf root stocks, with each dwarf apple tree expected to eventually produce 20 pounds of easy-to-harvest fruit."[9]

The City of Calgary is so serious about fruit production, that they are encouraging citizens to take up a hobby that has generated a bad buzz for American municipalities: beekeeping. Fruit trees need pollinators, and most varieties are pollinated by bees. Unfortunately, there has been a serious decline in honeybee populations throughout North America because of a number of factors, such as liberal pesticide use, climate change, loss of habitat, and predatory mites. In conjunction with the fruit tree plantings, the Urban Forestry Division introduced native mason bees at each orchard site to ensure pollination. (Mason bees, unlike honeybees, are solitary and nonaggressive. They will sting, but only as a response to being squeezed or stepped on.) The City even published an informational brochure teaching homeowners a simple, step-by-step process to build houses for mason bees.[10] Calgary's community orchard pilot program ended in 2014, so I asked Spence what her thoughts were. She said the program was a success. Spence learned quite a bit during the five-year pilot. Pears, for example, fared quite poorly in Calgary's climate. Some varieties had a zero survivability rate. But apples, cherries, and hazelnuts did quite well. She also learned that orchards that are planted in parks without an associative community group don't thrive like those planted in parks where there is already a large contingent of community gardeners. When you already have a group of people in the area gardening, they naturally look after the orchards. These gardeners prune, thin, harvest, and keep pests away. The trees in the stand-alone park, the one without any community association tied to it, saw heavy damage from deer and low fruit yields. Spence also sees a great opportunity to use the orchards as teaching tools. Parks staff train citizens on how to prune the trees and thin for higher fruit yields. Citizens then train other citizens. The result is healthy public fruit trees maintained by citizens without financial burden on city staff.

I asked Spence about the future of community orchards in Calgary, especially amid perennial concerns over lean municipal budgets. Spence said, "Funding is always a matter of prioritizing. Community orchards are community gathering places, and we listen to our community. These orchards are a priority."

Provo provides public vegetables and Calgary offers public fruits. In the central Ohio town of Worthington, one elected official says both are needed for community well-being.

City Councilman Doug Smith is pioneering *transitional* gardens in Worthington—a strategy to make the community happier, stronger, and more resilient in the face of a potentially fragile environment. *Transition* initiatives are responses to the challenges of an uncertain climate, economy, and resource supply. And public fruits and vegetables, in Councilman Smith's eyes, are resources that can help folks get by a little easier.

But Smith doesn't necessarily envision fruit trees planted like commercial orchards or vegetables replacing petunias outside of City Hall. Rather, Smith sees an opportunity to work with nature to allow underutilized public space throughout the city to feed folks, with little effort expended from staff. "The idea is to allow nature to 'do its thing' with minimal attention from the community and minimal resources from the city," said Smith. "Worthington is the perfect community in central Ohio to begin a transitional garden. We have public space that can sustain edible plants, and a lot of residents are happy to participate to increase community sustainability."[11]

This means planting mulberry, serviceberry, walnut, hickory, and pawpaw trees, because these species are native to central Ohio. And it means planting them in wooded thickets and along river banks, because these are the native habitats of these plants. The result is a large network of food-bearing plants that thrive because they are perfectly suited for their location.

The first phase of Smith's idea was completed in 2013, when

the City mapped the existing fruit and nut trees in town. Residents can simply go online and navigate a Google map to find local raspberries, walnuts, pawpaws, and apples. The website also helps residents with fruits they may not be familiar with. What are serviceberries, for example? A lot like blueberries, only a bit sweeter and mealier. You can eat them fresh from the bush, or you can visit the Worthington Resource Site to find recipes for serviceberry jam, spicy serviceberries, and serviceberry relish.[12] Providing information about serviceberries along with recipes takes the mystery out of this native-but-now-forgotten fruit, and it gets folks excited to forage for these new flavors.

The next phase of Smith's transitional gardens will be to plant more trees and shrubs throughout the city. Sure, seeding your public spaces with food helps feed people at little cost to the municipality. This is certainly a great benefit to the community. But Smith sees another great value of the public produce. For him, transitional gardens provide "a start to a long-term culture shift in Worthington to be closer to nature."

Across the continent, folks are demanding ready access to fresh, locally grown produce. It is becoming apparent that in the near future, municipalities will need to address urban agriculture as an important component of urban infrastructure, much like housing, transportation, and education. By simply allowing, encouraging, and implementing food gardens in public space, cities can meet that public demand, and in a fiscally responsible manner. Some municipal officials—like those in Provo, Calgary, and Worthington—have already recognized this, and have taken an active approach in the management of food-producing efforts in public space. These communities have proven that public parks, wooded river banks, and even the grounds around city hall are fantastic places to cultivate fruits and vegetables.

Though attitudes are changing, most public agencies discourage or downright prohibit the planting of edibles in these public

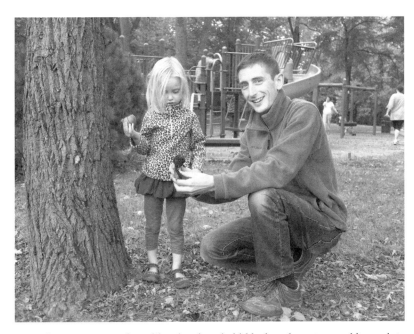

Councilman Doug Smith and his daughter hold black walnuts in a public park in Worthington, Ohio.

spaces, largely over concerns about maintenance and perceived mess. (Such judgments are often based on misperceptions, which will be addressed in greater detail in chapter 5.) These attitudes are especially prevalent with regard to city streets, which is quite unfortunate. Streets represent the largest, most extensive network of public space in cities, and thus are significant places to explore edible landscaping, as every person in every neighborhood could be reached. Along many streets, there is a boulevard or planting strip between the sidewalk and curb. Some streets are even outfitted with wide, landscaped medians down their center. Historically regarded as aesthetic enhancements to streets, these landscaped areas are proving fundamental to the popular "Green Streets" movement, which is being implemented in cities like New York, Seattle, and Portland. Using landscaping to capture stormwater runoff, thereby reducing pollution of our lakes, streams, and rivers, green streets also help moderate air temperature, improve air quality, and provide habitat for urban wildlife. Boulevards and medians offer great potential for incorporating food-bearing plants in the streetscape, especially fruit- and nut-bearing trees and shrubs. Not only are these larger plants desired to help define the street, and give neighborhoods character, but they can more quickly and efficiently transpire larger amounts of stormwater runoff. Incorporating agriculture along our streets helps communities attain broad equitable and environmental goals.

The City of Portland, Oregon, is one municipality that does recognize the food-producing potential of city streets. Staff in that municipality's Parks and Recreation Department are seeking to codify the acceptance of fruit trees for their use as street trees. Persimmon, Asian pear, pear, and fig are handsome trees that can spruce up any street, while also providing delicious and nutritious food. Though such a policy falls short of hearty encouragement to plant food-bearing trees in the public right-of-way, at least it absolves the owner of crime (or guilt) for wanting to establish some form of public food production. Even if public officials do not follow Portland's lead and cannot be convinced to allow fruit and nut trees along public streets, medians and boulevards still present excellent opportunities to plant smaller, tidier crops such as blueberries, dwarf citrus, strawberries, herbs, and annual vegetables.

While streets are the most extensive network of public space, the most concentrated and diverse group of public sites is found downtown. Plazas, town squares, courtyards, parks, streets, parking lots, and various civic buildings proliferate in the urban core of our cities. Coincidentally, downtowns have become the largest food deserts in our communities. Sure, there is a plethora of cafés, restaurants, and sandwich shops, but good luck finding fresh, locally grown, organic, and *cheap* fruits and vegetables. Downtowns are thus ideal for exploring the benefits of public produce.

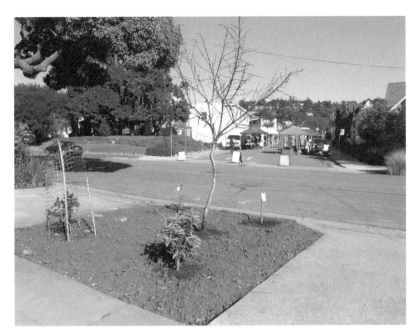

In this generous space between the sidewalk and curb, a modest orchard has just been planted: Comice pear, apricot, Meyer lemon, and clementine surround an already established cherry tree. Of course, being across the street from the local farmers' market helps instill the desire for fresh, local produce.

Of course, microclimatic conditions can be challenging downtown, with high-rise buildings casting deep shade over some areas throughout much of the day—not to mention the turbulent wind tunnels that are often experienced within the urban canyons of downtown. Downtown buildings also generate and reflect a lot of heat, creating a heat island that, while disadvantageous in some respects, especially with regard to energy use, could be beneficial for urban agriculture in northern cities. Annual vegetables, for example, can often be started earlier—and extend later into the growing season—when planted downtown, because temperatures tend to be warmer than in more remote, less-developed parts of the city. In general, the planting of gardens downtown should be encouraged,

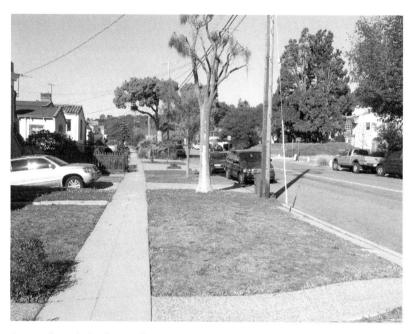

A typical sterile landscape that the owners obviously dread maintaining.

as gardens help improve air quality and moderate temperature, absorb stormwater, and provide much-needed greenery, softening the
hard surfaces of the concrete canyons. The trick is to find those
public spaces where even the most micro of microclimates is con-
ducive to growing food. There are plenty.

Downtowns commonly possess another type of prevalent space:
the vacant lot. As I mentioned, folks tending crops on vacant lots
is often the image we conjure when we think of urban agriculture.
While the use of vacant lots to grow food can be an integral component of a successful network of public produce, these parcels are not
what we typically think of as public space—the sorts of places where
concentrations of diverse people stroll through or gather together to
recreate, socialize, or simply pass the time. These lots are "public"
merely because they have been abandoned, leaving the municipality
with no choice but to assume ownership. In function, abandoned

property is not public space—just simple open space. But this type of open-space cultivation does share some civic benefits with more traditional public space, namely, helping to build community.

The argument for vacant lot cultivation is quite sensible: it allows land that nobody is interested in developing (at the time) to return to productive use, while lessening visual blight and bolstering community pride. Some community gardens have even helped to reduce crime in troubled neighborhoods and have raised property values of adjacent structures. These obvious benefits give rise to an ironic new problem: by effectively mitigating blight, the successful community garden on a vacant lot increases the appeal of a dilapidated neighborhood, and that, in turn, increases development interest. In the minds of many public officials, community gardens on vacant lots serve only as placeholders until a developer is interested in improving the property. But to the community, the garden is a source of pride and good food, with years of sweat and toil poured into the soil. Raze the gardens to build homes, and you raise frustrations citizens have toward their government.

Such a situation is exactly what happened in New York during the late 1990s. New York City had a long list of active community gardens, some dating back to the early 1970s. Many in the community revered these green spaces, but to NYC public officials, those garden sites were merely placeholders for future housing. In May 1998, Mayor Rudolph Giuliani transferred hundreds of community garden sites from the city's Parks Department to the Department of Housing Preservation and Development. This seemingly benign act spelled imminent doom for the gardens, as the policy opinions of Parks staff are very different from Housing and Development staff. To help generate revenue, the city's Office of Management and Budget mandated that the garden sites be either developed or auctioned. Mayor Giuliani's administration argued that the gardens were never meant to be permanent. The community argued otherwise, and a bitter green-bean war ensued. Protesters dressed as fruits and vegetables rallied outside the mayor's office, newspapers joined the fray and seemed to side with the gardeners, while Mayor Giuliani taunted, "Welcome to the era after communism."[13]

In the end, 113 garden sites were spared from development, but at a hefty cost. Trust for Public Land and New York Restoration, a community-based land trust led by entertainer Bette Midler, purchased the properties from the city for $4.2 million. Community groups declared victory, but, as one garden group noted, "forcing supporters of community gardens to pay the City millions of dollars to secure a future for community gardeners is bad public policy."[14] As New York and other municipalities across the country have learned, using community gardens as economic placeholders for future development is proving to be an unpopular strategy. If a garden site is successful, and has a group of dedicated citizens bent on improving the neighborhood and the lives of its inhabitants, it can be political suicide to try to take that land away.

What if community gardens were to make money? If urban agriculture was deemed a viable business to a plucky entrepreneur, would the city's stance on vacant-land cultivation change? University of Wisconsin professors Jerry Kaufman and Martin Bailkey sought to answer that question, and studied the extent to which entrepreneurial urban agriculture could be established on abandoned property in America. The impetus of their report is intriguing, as they cite the tens of thousands of vacant properties in each of the cities of Milwaukee, St. Louis, New Orleans, Chicago, Detroit, and Philadelphia that could reclaim productivity while establishing food security for these cities' food-poor citizens. The examples of the many urban agricultural efforts being attempted within various communities was heartening evidence of a nascent, national trend. In the end, however, Kaufman and Bailkey concluded their analysis with the realization that "city government leaders would like their middle-class residents to stay instead of moving to the suburbs. They wish for more market housing and small businesses located on vacant land. They would like to see a strong back-to-the-city movement to help fuel revitalization of depressed neighborhoods."[15] The pair could not find much support for their ideas even from venerable, farsighted planners like Edmund Bacon. Their report recounted an argument Bacon made to the *Philadelphia Daily News* on his ninetieth birthday. Bacon urged planners and public officials to "wake up" to the amount of land that has been abandoned in their cities, and to find more rational uses for that land. Urban agriculture was not the rational use Bacon proffered, however. Instead, his strategy was to clear all vacant houses in order to assemble large tracts of obstruction-free land, which could entice housing developers to build new neighborhoods.[16]

Kaufman and Bailkey reasonably argue that the middle-class exodus continues in many American cities, and that considerable property—particularly that without the virtue of being near the city center or along a waterfront—will remain vacant and unsightly for the foreseeable future. Surely, in these areas, entrepreneurial urban agriculture makes good planning sense.

Such is the case in Detroit, a city estimated to have forty square miles of vacant land—30 percent of the city's total area. In the 1950s, Detroit's population was almost two million. Sixty years later, over 60 percent of that former population has fled, creating the largest urban population decline in American history. With the massive depopulation, the City of Detroit inherited tens of thousands of vacant parcels. Community groups have been turning many of these vacant parcels into food-growing opportunities for over a decade, and their efforts have inspired many. In some ways, Detroit is the embodiment of the National Vacant Properties Campaign slogan, "Creating opportunity from abandonment."[17] Now, thoughts are moving beyond the community garden plot to larger farming efforts. Some would like to see Detroit turn eyesore into opportunity by becoming the greenest city in the nation. Indeed, many urban planners see this bounty of empty land as a literal blank slate, with fantastic potential to reinvent Detroit. But even with all the vacant land, with more likely to come, and amid projections that it would take at least an entire generation before

Detroit could be repopulated, policy makers still pine for the days when Detroit peaked at two million people. The thought of plants taking up space that could be inhabited by houses is a tough pill for some to swallow.[18]

Efforts to reinvent Detroit through urban agriculture give reason to believe that vacant lot cultivation in other cities is a worthy revitalization strategy. However, many city planners and policy makers will likely continue to align with the planning strategy offered by Edmund Bacon. There is no denying the potential beauty and communal good that is possible with vacant lot cultivation. But when there is an opportunity (or even hope) to bolster the tax base, create real density and diversity in the community, and revitalize a neighborhood with new homes and businesses, urban agriculture will seldom be seen as the highest and best use of abandoned land.

If a community insists on continued cultivation of vacant land in the face of a reluctant municipality, one option is to enlist the assistance of a land trust. Land trusts will acquire and hold land in perpetuity for the purpose of protecting that land from development.[19] There are many types of land trusts organized for many different purposes. Chicago's NeighborSpace, in particular, provides a unique land-trust model for municipally supported urban agriculture.

NeighborSpace is a community-based, intergovernmental partnership between the City of Chicago, Chicago Parks District, and the Forest Preserve District of Cook County. Staff from each of these local agencies serve on NeighborSpace's board of directors, and each government partner commits $100,000 annually to acquire titles to vacant land, which they then deed to community groups who spare that land from development. There are many reasons to protect land from development, such as environmental conservation, historic preservation, land assembly for real estate speculation, and recreation, to name a few. What makes NeighborSpace unique is its pledge to "committed neighbors (who) have come together to turn vacant lots, railway, river embankments, and other open space into gardens and parks for community food production and beautification."[20] While many NeighborSpace sites are used for parks and ornamental gardens, protecting sites for the production of food is becoming more commonplace. It is this commitment to food production on urban open space and the active involvement and financial investment of local government officials that give promise to the tenure of urban agriculture on abandoned property.

Land trusts like NeighborSpace generally have excellent track records of successfully securing land for the preservation of open space, but there are times when an opponent proves too formidable. NeighborSpace was unsuccessful with one irregularly shaped, city-owned parcel on North Sheffield Avenue in Chicago. It was not the municipality that objected to the proposal for an urban agriculture demonstration project, but the neighborhood. Residents overwhelmingly felt that the site's highest and best use was housing. In what was certainly a rare example of NIMBYism (a derivative of the acronym for "Not In My Back Yard"), one that might provoke incredulity from many urban planners, neighbors argued that the community's appearance would be best improved not with green space, but with a building.[21]

There will always be controversy over what constitutes the highest and best use of abandoned property in struggling neighborhoods. During prolonged periods of economic woe, development declines sharply and hunger rises. Growing food for people is arguably the best use for land that lies fallow during such times. Indeed, it often takes such catastrophic collapses for public officials to reassess their public policies. While a few ardent activists have perennially advocated for better options in public transportation, for example, such pleas have historically fallen on deaf ears—until the price of gasoline leaped above four dollars per gallon.

Such is the case with urban agriculture. As we have moved into uncertain economic and climatic times, public officials across the country have taken notice of the nation's fragile food supply. The interest in growing food on vacant land to help establish food security has not been this strong since the victory garden effort of

World War II. But history has taught us a lesson: the economy is cyclical, and we will witness prosperity again. And when those jubilant times come hence, the land that once lay fallow—that no one but gardeners and food growers would touch—will become, once again, prime for development. As long as municipalities maintain control over vacant land, or uphold zoning regulations that restrict property to certain types of development, urban agriculture efforts on abandoned parcels will continue to be ephemeral. Only when the municipality relinquishes control of the land, or a long-term lease is agreed upon, will longevity be guaranteed to the community garden.

What could be a more permanent and acceptable strategy—to both citizens and public officials—is to look to other forms of public space in the city for urban agriculture. In any city, there are numerous underutilized public and open spaces that could be used to produce food. According to Luc Mougeot, an expert on urban agriculture efforts around the world, "municipal governments that have mapped their city's open spaces are amazed by how much space sits idle at any given time." He further contends that "unused urban space is a wasted opportunity—an asset denied to a community's well-being and a brake on the city's development."[22]

Mougeot believes that urban agriculture strategies perform best when they can be retrofitted onto public and open spaces where other activities are already occurring. "Setting aside areas in or around the city for the exclusive and permanent use by urban agriculture is unrealistic and self-defeating," he argues. "For one thing, it ignores the economic reality of land prices in growing cities. More importantly, it misses out on the interactions that urban agriculture can have (and should have, if it is to prosper) with other urban activities." Instead, Mougeot urges municipal government to take a critical look at the myriad public and open spaces, and to ask probing questions, such as, "How much space in their city is unused, underused, or misused? Where? How much of this could be made more attractive, more productive, and more profitable in social, economic, and environmental terms? How much could be achieved, in the short or longer term, through urban agriculture?"[23] Public spaces that are too large for the density of the surrounding development (suburban parks and parking lots); too uncomfortable or uninteresting to attract a sufficient number of users (many downtown plazas); or where development is either not possible or not allowed (street rights-of-way, floodplains, utility and transportation easements) provide great alternative sites to vacant lot cultivation. And these urban spaces, as they are tucked in and around our places of employment, commerce, recreation, and residence, provide that interaction of urban activities that Mougeot believes is necessary in our cities.

The City of Chicago has recently done exactly what Mougeot has advised, by mapping their underutilized land. And what they determined was that with so much fallow real estate, there is room for both development and agriculture. The city of Chicago believes there's a great future for cultivating much of this land, for the sake of its citizens' health and the city's financial well-being. The city has adopted a pioneering program dubbed "Farmers for Chicago," which aggregates as much as five acres of vacant land per farming activity on the South Side. Mayor Rahm Emanuel believes, "Once made available, these vacant lots will help stabilize communities by bringing productive activity to areas that need it around food deserts."[24]

Mayor Emanuel's program is a manifestation of the broader but equally pioneering food policy "Eat Local Live Healthy." This prior policy, adopted by Emanuel's predecessor Mayor Richard M. Daley, identifies "food issues that, if restructured locally, could improve food quality, lower its cost and increase its availability for consumers."[25] Authored by the municipality's Department of Planning and Development, Eat Local Live Healthy outlines a framework of strategies that not only enhance public health but create food-related business opportunities and foster public- and private-sector cooperation. Increasing food production in Chicago neighborhoods; improving access to locally grown, healthful food; and boosting public awareness of the availability and benefits of locally sourced food are just a few of the strategies outlined in Eat Local Live Healthy.

Cities like Chicago are ripe to take the next step in offering choices in locally sourced food on public land. And if the folks at City Hall are going to lead by example, then there is no better, more symbolic place to showcase public produce than City Hall itself.

While visiting Germany in 2000, Mayor Daley witnessed various aspects of urban agriculture and was reportedly inspired to implement some of these efforts back home in the Windy City. An incredible opportunity for local food production was found right under his nose, or more specifically, over his head. Today, on the northwest corner of City Hall's roof, a colony of over 200,000 honeybees is churning out sweet rewards for this municipality's local food philosophy.

In 2003, shortly after construction was completed for City Hall's "green roof"—a garden in the sky that helps to insulate the building, reduce stormwater runoff, moderate air temperature, and provide habitat for butterflies and migratory birds—Daley asked two beekeepers from a local honey co-op to erect an apiary. Two hives of Italian honeybees were installed by Stephanie Averill and Michael Thompson, who manage the apiary and harvest its crop. The bees pollinate flowers as far as five miles from City Hall, returning with nectar to produce two seasonal—and two very distinct—blends of honey. During the spring and summer, the bulk of the nectar is collected from white clover, yielding a very light honey with superior taste. In the autumn, goldenrod and white aster nectar produce a darker and richer honey crop, better used for cooking. The honey, which is sold at the Chicago Cultural Center, the City of Chicago Store, and through the Internet is proving popular with locals and visitors alike. The proceeds from honey sales are funneled into the municipality's Department of Cultural Affairs to help support free public programs, such as art exhibits, performances, and other cultural events.

The city's honey program has been so successful that more hives were placed atop other city buildings. Michael Thompson noted that four hives were added to the green roof at the Chicago Cultural Center and two atop the green roof at Gallery 37 Center for the Arts.[26] Chicago's green roofs provide a sterling example of the immense value that can be extracted from a typically forgotten public space. And the honey that is produced and sold proves that buying local food is not only good for the environment but good for culture and community as well.[27]

In retrospect, Mayor Daley's directive to construct an apiary atop City Hall was prophetically visionary. As the City of Calgary learned when they planted an abundance of fruit trees but then witnessed a dearth of pollinators, nations today—particularly the United States and Canada—are grappling with the startling decline in the honeybee population, referred to as Colony Collapse Disorder (CCD). And with the decline in honeybee populations comes a decline in food production. Many vegetable, fruit, and nut crops require pollination from honey bees. Human existence, we are quickly learning, is thus inextricably linked to these busy little bugs. Without bees to pollinate our plants, CCD, as author Michael Shacker postulates, could well lead to "Civilization Collapse Disorder."[28] Treating honey bees as pests and controlling their population through insecticides is endangering the health of plants, the planet, and all of its inhabitants. Municipalities nationwide should follow Chicago's (and Calgary's) lead and erect apiaries to do their part to encourage active, productive bee colonies. While CCD is still a mystery, and entomologists work feverishly to find its cause, the best we can do to end this syndrome is garden organically, and to take up beekeeping in our city spaces, so we can better understand—and appreciate—our wild pollinators.

Chicago is unique in its comprehensive, top-down approach to food security. The mayors of this progressive city, both past and present, advocate for sweeping and reformative food policies that have typically been lobbied for by grassroots groups. It seems these mayors truly understand the relationship between food security, community health, and economic prosperity, and are pioneering strategies to ensure that citizens have access to local, fresh food. In his introductory letter to Eat Local Live Healthy, Mayor Daley explains, "Local and fresh food would be most beneficial to our health, environment, and economy. But much of the produce we buy comes from places like California, Chile or New Zealand. There are global environmental costs of shipping produce so far. And, the farther it is shipped, the less fresh it can be."[29]

What this great city succinctly illustrates is that public produce is an amalgam of public space, public officials, and public policy. If public produce is to be truly effective in bolstering the health and well-being of the city's citizens, municipalities must lead by example. Mayor Daley in particular recognized that commodity crops such as corn and soy bolster the city's economy, but they do not feed people directly. He warned Chicagoans of the need to restructure the city's food system to provide access to healthy, local table food. What Daley sensibly advocated was greater food choices in the community, choices that improve both the health of his city's citizens and the health of his city's economy. Growing food on public land, as part of a broader food policy, can offer the choices Daley advocated for. Daley readily admitted that, given Chicago's northern climate, some food items will still have to be imported. But in a plain-spoken manner that only Midwesterners have mastered, using the sort of pragmatic logic that is difficult to argue with, Daley reasoned, "Importing some food is different from importing most of it."[30]

Chapter 4

To Glean and Forage in the City

When you reap the harvest of your land, you shall not reap all the way to the edges of your field, or gather the gleanings of your harvest. You shall not pick your vineyard bare, or gather the fallen fruit of your vineyard; you shall leave them for the poor and the stranger. Leviticus 19:9–10

A T THE END OF THE 2008 GROWING SEASON, a farming couple outside of Denver opened their fields to anyone who wanted to gather potatoes, beets, carrots, and onions left over from the harvest. The Millers, owners of the farm, had never made such an offer before, but thought it could be a way to thank their customers while ensuring that perfectly good food did not go to waste. They arranged for the public giveaway to begin at 9:00 a.m. on the Saturday before Thanksgiving, and put the word out to the local media, thinking that over the course of the weekend, five thousand people might take them up on their offer.

They underestimated.

Forty thousand people—the size of a small city—arrived at the Miller farm to gather free food. People began lining up before dawn. By 8:30 a.m., the Millers' five-acre parking lot was full, and they had to direct cars out onto the open fields. The line of cars waiting to pick fresh, free produce extended over two miles down Highway 66. At the end of the first day of what was supposed to be a two-day harvest, the fields were picked clean, and an estimated 600,000 pounds of produce went home to grateful families.[1]

The public response to the Millers' benevolent gesture reveals the hunger people have for fresh, free produce. "People obviously need food," noted Mrs. Miller.[2] Another woman thought it was the economic freefall in 2008 that spurred such a large response. "Everybody is so depressed about the economy. . . . This was a pure party. Everybody having a great time getting something for free."[3]

Perhaps the circumstances of the Great Recession did provoke the outpouring of people seeking fresh produce from the Millers' farm that day. But I believe there is more to unearth from this event than just people making a trek for free food. It was made clear to anybody wanting food from the Millers' farm that they would have to pick it from the fields themselves: to get down on the ground and get their hands dirty. I suspect if the Millers had instead offered to hand out sacks of onions and potatoes to anybody who showed up—in the manner of a food bank—the response would not have been as large. There can be a certain shame that accompanies the acceptance of handouts, as it invites pity. Working for one's meals, on the other hand, is respectable, and it may have been the opportunity for folks to labor for its rewards, rather than merely accepting charity, that provoked the large response.

More to the point, I believe it was the prospect of harvesting, the specific act of venturing out into the fields and pulling food from the earth—proof to one's self that one has the wherewithal to provide for the family—that provided as much compulsion for people that day as the food's gratis price tag, perhaps more so. The huge crowd that turned out to pick produce reflected the desire people have for a bit of agrarianism in their urban lifestyles.

The practice of gleaning—gathering food left over in the fields from the commercial harvest—is an age-old manner of putting food on the table. In many parts of the world, though, gleaning has long been stigmatized. While some consider it entirely appropriate (and perfectly respectable) to gather food that would otherwise rot, others see it as a pitiful endeavor, a practice undertaken only by those down on their luck.

The French realist painter Jean-François Millet sought to erase the stigma of gathering food left behind by others in his brilliant mid-nineteenth-century portrait *Les Glaneuses* (The Gleaners). Millet depicts a melancholy scene: peasant women, in the twilight of the day, their backs hunched over the harvested fields of rural France, collecting leftover grains that lay on the ground with their dirty, masculine hands. Yet, Millet expertly portrays an air of dignity within the scene. The subjects are gleaners after all, not beggars, and there is pride in an honest day's toil. These women, though they stoop for scraps, are not to be pitied. They ably provide for themselves and their families.

Gleaning persists in France to this day, and a provocative film *The Gleaners and I* documents how this practice has evolved over the last 150 years. Producer Agnès Varda builds on the dignity depicted in Millet's portrait, poignantly illustrating how gleaning continues to be a respectable method of providing for the family. But women are no longer the sole gleaners, as was depicted in Millet's portrait and in others painted at the time. Men and children now commonly glean the fields of France.[4]

Varda focuses on the myriad groups that still benefit from gleaning —from today's rural peasants to urban artists. Restaurateurs are some of the more intriguing beneficiaries of leftover produce. One subject, a gourmet chef, gleans simply because of the steep

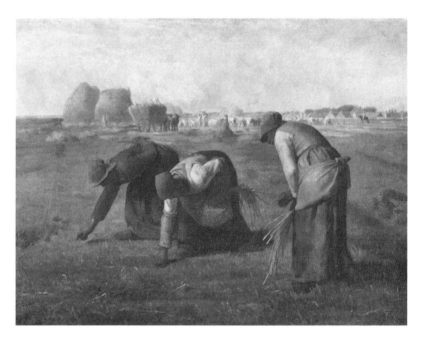

Jean-François Millet's Les Glaneuses (The Gleaners), *1857.*

overhead of the restaurant business, and survival requires frugality. The chef, at the time the youngest in France to have received two stars from the esteemed Michelin Guide, laments the huge price that savory and other fresh herbs command. To combat the rising cost of quality ingredients, he roams the nearby fields in the morning, picking and gleaning what is necessary for the day's menu. Not only does this save his restaurant money, but it gives him an assurance of quality: he knows exactly from where and when the produce was harvested.

For this same reason, other subjects in Varda's film glean hundreds of pounds of potatoes to sell to restaurants looking for fresh, locally grown produce at an attractive price. Some of these potatoes are nicked or blemished, or too misshapen to be saleable in any market. Others are simply too large. Only those potatoes that are of a certain caliber and complexion are delivered to market;

all others—about twenty-five tons—are dumped in the fields to rot because consumers supposedly will not waste good money on homely produce. Restaurateurs, however, always look for ways to trim the price of quality ingredients, and they buy the gleaned potatoes by the bushels. It does not matter what the potatoes look like to the restaurateur, because after he or she is done with them, nobody will know that they were once ugly. For chefs, what matters most are flavor, texture, and freshness. Even though these potatoes at one time looked unpalatable to the markets, they are just as flavorful and texturally rich as their more handsome siblings.

Varda's film reveals that gleaning is still practiced—and even relished—by many in rural France. The hordes that pulled up at the Miller farm suggest Americans crave opportunities to gather food as well. But the real proof of our yearning to regrow our agrarian roots is the success of U-Pick farms—a business that, until recently, would be as profitable as selling sea water to a sailor.

It seems a bit absurd that many of us drive an hour (or longer) to an orchard and pay farmers for the opportunity to harvest their fruit for them. Surely if we wanted orchard-fresh produce, a quick trip to the local farmers' market could sate our craving. But it doesn't. Buying produce from a farmers' market, though more soulfully enriching than a trip to Safeway or Kroger, is still a simple consumer transaction. Farmers' markets don't offer the connection to nature, or the sense of self-sufficiency, that pulling a potato from the dirt or plucking a pear from a tree offers. Yes, it is absurd that agri-tourism is now a profitable industry. But it is more absurd that we no longer have opportunities to pick produce in our own communities.

Or do we? Gail Savina says, indeed, the opportunity to pluck food straight from nature's hand is right under our noses. Or more accurately, above our heads.

Savina is the founder of City Fruit, a Seattle not-for-profit bent on reclaiming the urban orchard. City Fruit believes urban fruit is a valuable community resource, but a resource that is squandered because few know how to harvest all the food, or what to do with the entire bounty once they have it in their hands. One common scenario goes something like this: Homeowners get giddy over the thought of planting a fruit tree in their yard, because who doesn't want fresh plums from time to time? Except we forget just how prolific a single plum tree can be. We eat a few fresh plums, but there are so many more left. What to do? Well, we can always make a plum cobbler. Except we don't really know how to cook. Ooh! We can try making plum jam! But our grandmother never showed us how, and the recipes on the Internet look complicated. Well, maybe we can just eat a few more fresh plums. Before we know it, we've had our fill of plums for the year, and the rest fall to the ground with a squish.

And now the other scenario: Renters buy their first home with a nice yard. "Oh Honey, isn't it just lovely? Look, it even has an apple tree!" But lo and behold, that tree turned out to be a heavy-bearing apple tree. These renters-turned-homeowners don't bake, don't need or want to eat that many apples (though they love the romantic notion of having an apple tree in the backyard), and suddenly have a headache on their hands.

What to do with our fruit surplus is an annual dilemma for most of us. For Seattleites, they have City Fruit. Landowners (including the City of Seattle) simply register their fruit trees with Savina's organization, and when the fruit is ripe, City Fruit will send out a harvesting crew and pick the fruit for free. This is a huge benefit to fruit tree owners, as they are freed from the hassles of disposing of unwanted fruit. But it is a huge benefit for the community as well.

In 2013, City Fruit gleaned 8,500 pounds of fruit from 135 sites; 7,000 pounds were donated to local food banks and meal programs, and the remaining 1,500 pounds were sold to Seattle restaurants, generating over $3,000 in revenue. When Savina told me that the fanciest restaurants in Seattle bought her urban fruit, it surprised me at first. But then I remembered that restaurateurs love gleaned produce, because they know the food is fresh and the provenance is sterling. And for Seattle's many eco-conscious chefs concerned with food miles, this fruit is as local as it gets.

I asked Savina how she determines what gets donated and what gets sold to restaurants. She said it was quite easy. As it turns out, the fruits chefs prize are the fruits food banks have little need for. "Food banks want the more mainstream, less fragile stuff, like apples, pears, plums, and grapes," Savina explained. "But we also harvest figs, quince, crabapples, and persimmon. Restaurants love these, as they are always looking for unique ingredients."[5]

In addition to gleaning from private trees,[6] City Fruit also developed a community stewardship program to care for public fruit trees. According to City Fruit's website, over thirty Seattle parks have fruit trees—many of these vestiges of farmstead orchards. Not only do these heritage trees continue to yield good fruit, but they bolster the urban forest and are a link to Seattle's past. Unfortunately, the Parks Department lacks the staff to properly care for these holdovers. Parks will do larger-scale pruning from time to time. But they can't do the sorts of things that fruit trees require for serious fruit production, like biannual pruning, fruit thinning, and harvesting. So City Fruit, with financial assistance from Washington State's Department of Natural Resources and Seattle's Parks Department, assigns orchard stewards for these specialized tasks. This guarantees these old trees thrive while coaxing more food from those historic branches, ensuring that Seattleites can thrive as well.[7]

Gleaning groups like City Fruit are rapidly sprouting across the country. Solid Ground gleans fruit trees in Seattle neighborhoods that City Fruit cannot get to. The mission for Los Angeles's Food Forward can be summed up in one word: fruitanthropy (which the group defines as the picking and donating of fruit for humanitarian purposes).[8] Unlike other public gleaning groups, Food Forward gleans vegetables as well (veggianthropy?). In the four years they've been operating, the group has gleaned a whopping 1.9 million pounds of urban produce! The Baltimore Orchard Project not only gleans fruit from existing trees, but plants community orchards, too. Most can only fantasize about the types of fruit Maui's Waste Not, Want Not foundation gleans from neighborhood trees: Bananas, litchis, tangerines, mangoes, avocados, breadfruit, oranges, limes, and pineapples; lots and lots of pineapples. How much is a lot? Some 400,000 pounds per year, according to the group's website.[9]

Gleaning fresh produce from our own community is praiseworthy. But it is also lots of fun. The reason these local organizations are able to glean 10,000 pounds of apples (or 400,000 pounds of pineapples!) each year is because of the hundreds of volunteers a harvesting opportunity attracts. Of course, the mission of these gleaning groups is inspiring. But so is the mission of countless other charities who struggle to attract volunteers. Picking fruit—whether for ourselves or others—lightens our mood and lifts our spirit. The Portland Fruit Tree Project calls their gleaning events "harvesting *parties*," because that is really what they are: groups of people getting together for a merry time over food. As one volunteer fruitanthropist for L.A.'s Food Forward noted, "I really didn't expect fruit picking to be so fun, but it was! It's hard not to feel the stress of the day melt away as you laugh about getting bopped on the head by a small citrus fruit, or feeling satisfied climbing high into a tree to pick the freshest grapefruit for someone in need."[10]

While neighborhood gleaning is a more convenient (and eco-friendly, and maybe even fun) manner of getting our agrarian fix than driving a few dozen miles to a U-Pick farm, there is one significant limitation: access. As you may have discerned, the overwhelming bulk of the fruit harvested from these gleaning groups comes from privately owned trees. This means going into someone's backyard (and obtaining their permission before doing so), just to pluck a few pears. If you're picking because you just want to do something great for your community, volunteering with neighborhood gleaning groups on the weekend is a fantastic opportunity. But what if you want a few cherries just for yourself? On a Wednesday, maybe, for a dessert you wish to make. Or maybe you

realize you are out of apples for your child's lunch. You could sub-
stitute oranges, except you know what's coming . . . "But Daa-aad!
I really want APPLES!" The farmers' market was last night, and you
really don't want to wait in line at the supermarket. You want to be
able to walk down your street or through your neighborhood park
to harvest the fruit you need—freely, without restriction or permission. You want opportunities to truly forage in your city.

In Los Angeles, a creative organization known as Fallen Fruit pro-
motes social equity, public health, and environmental stewardship
through the act of foraging for fruit. Though they roam neighborhoods and pick fruit just like other urban gleaning organizations,
Fallen Fruit's harvests have one notable distinction: they are all
done from public space.

The group, founded by three Los Angeles artists, unearthed an
arcane city ordinance—a usufruct law—that states that fruits over-
hanging any public space, regardless of whether the tree is planted
on private property or not, are public goods. In general usage, usufruct laws give a person legal access to somebody else's property,
provided that the property is not damaged. What this means in
the city of Los Angeles is that fruits that can be plucked from city
sidewalks, parks, and even semipublic spaces like parking lots and
plazas where permission to pass is granted to the public, are considered fair game, and protected by law.

So the three artists would roam their neighborhoods and pick
fruit from the alleys and sidewalks. As word spread, others would
join the trio on their fruit forays. And for a different experience,
the group would sometimes harvest at night. Though their fruit
harvests were protected by law, harvesting in the dark blurred the
line between public and private space, lawful and unlawful fruit,
adding more thrill to the picking. (You know artists; it's always
about raw emotion.)

But then the group did something quite ingenious: they started
drawing neighborhood maps locating all the fruit trees with

publicly accessible branches. Color-coded star shapes pinpoint the location of avocados and kumquats on Murietta, for example, or the tangerines and lemons on Albers. By drawing maps and posting them on their website, they made it possible for *anyone* to amble through the neighborhoods of Los Angeles and pick fruit, whenever they wanted. These maps gave the forager freedom compared to gleaning groups, who tell you where to harvest and when.

The maps, quite arresting in their simplicity, convey a lot of information. Not only do they identify all the fruit trees in each neighborhood and where to find them, but each map includes a legend denoting when each type of fruit is in season: guavas and prickly pear in spring; figs, bananas, and plums in summer; avocados and citrus year-round. And each map includes friendly, pithy advice, reminding foragers to "take only what you need, share your food, take a friend and say 'Hi' to strangers."

Even more ingenious is that these maps are a sort of wiki database of the world's public fruit. If you want to map the trees in your neighborhood, Fallen Fruit provides the graphic template. Simply follow their format, identify and map the trees, and return the map to Fallen Fruit. Your map will then be added to their website along with the ever-expanding catalog of fruit tree maps in other communities.

The mapping idea took off. Soon, public fruit maps were created for cities all over the country: San Francisco, Santa Fe, Boulder, and Virginia City. And then the idea went global. Log on to Fallen Fruit's website today, and you will see fruit maps of Copenhagen, Malmö, Guadalajara, and Madrid. These maps have given Fallen Fruit international acclaim. And it is well deserved. The simple, sublime act of mapping a neighborhood's fruit trees has forced us to recognize the great community resource that urban fruit is.

In his revelatory book *The Omnivore's Dilemma*, Michael Pollan sought to better answer the age-old question, "What should we have for dinner?" After traipsing through the cornfields of Iowa;

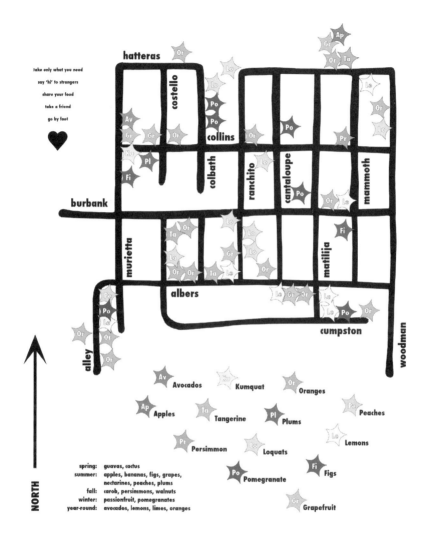

FALLEN FRUIT OF SHERMAN OAKS

The Fallen Fruit map of the Sherman Oaks neighborhood of Los Angeles, locating the different fruit trees with publicly accessible fruit. The map provides a code to the seasons in which the fruits are ready for harvest. Each map also bears the mantra: "take only what you need, say 'hi' to strangers, share your food, take a friend, go by foot."

chicken ranches in Virginia; and feedlots, food science laboratories, and organic mega-ranches throughout the country, he finds himself back at home in the Bay Area, on a quest to find dessert. Pollan recollects:

> My plan was to forage fruit, for a tart, from one of the many fruit trees lining the streets in Berkeley. I see no reason why foraging for food should be restricted to the countryside, so . . . I embarked on several urban scouting expeditions in quest of dessert. Actually, these were just strolls around the neighborhood with a baggie. In the two years we've lived in Berkeley I've located a handful of excellent fruit trees—plum, apple, apricot, and fig—offering publicly accessible branches.[11]

Having lived in Berkeley for many years myself, I can attest to the bounty of food-producing shrubs and trees that line the neighborhood streets. In addition to those that Pollan had found, I have seen oranges, lemons, cherries, persimmon, fennel, the occasional tomato vine, as well as rosemary, thyme, sage, and other herbs—all occupying space between the sidewalk and the street. Though these plants may have been purchased and planted by private homeowners, their location in the public right-of-way means they now belong to everybody. In short, it is entirely plausible to find dessert—and more—merely by strolling the streets of Berkeley.

Pollan's quest to forage in the city was more than a conceit. While he admits gathering entire meals from one's urban surrounds is probably not feasible on a regular basis, he believes it is an important endeavor undertaken occasionally to remind us where our food comes from. Much of the food security problems plaguing the nation today stem from this lack of knowledge, Pollan argues. Understanding what fruits and vegetables can grow in your community, and when they are ready to eat, offers many benefits, not the least of which is the personal challenge to provide for oneself and succeed, providing satiety for both the body and spirit.

Surely one can learn about the nature and culture of eating, as Pollan hoped to do foraging for ingredients for his fruit tart. But gathering food from your community can also yield more tangible benefits. Not only is it more eco-friendly to harvest fresh produce locally rather than having it trucked in from a distant region, but gathering food can supplement caloric intake by providing nourishment in the form of snacks, or on occasion, complete meals. For children, being able to forage for fresh produce in the city may mean the difference between a bag of chips on the way home from school or an apple. For the working poor, foraging may mean the difference between skipping meals in order to pay the electric bill or a healthy dinner. And for the utterly destitute, foraging may mean the difference between food from a public plaza or a dumpster. Public produce can help those hit hardest by the rising cost of fresh food, or those who do not have ready access to it.

American cities today are grappling with a shrinking middle class and a growing number of have-nots, particularly in the wake of our last recession. Hunger is usually—and erroneously—associated with the down-and-out, such as the homeless. The truth is, hunger can afflict all walks of life. As the San Francisco–Marin Food Bank reminds us, "High unemployment, a tough economy and the rising cost of living have pushed record numbers of people to the brink of hunger. Families who have always lived securely in the middle class are now seeking help at our food pantries."

The SF–Marin food bank provides an interesting snapshot of the growing numbers of people who are skipping dinner, eating less, or eating less well to make ends meet. In the one-million-person region of San Francisco and Marin counties, over 225,000 seek food assistance. That's one in four people. Only 14 percent of these almost quarter million individuals are homeless. The rest are seniors on fixed incomes, the middle-aged who recently lost their jobs, young adults working at low-wage jobs, and children. Many, many children.[12]

You're probably thinking, "Yeah, but that's San Francisco, one of the most expensive places to live in the world." Well, the situation is about as dire in the Heartland. Gleaners, a food bank serving central Indiana, notes that one in six Hoosiers can't get enough to eat either. And of the one million people they serve, one in three are children. While the numbers of Americans going without food are certainly alarming, Gleaners reminds us that food insecurity doesn't mean folks are perennially starving:

> Food insecurity means a lack of access, at times, to enough food for an active, healthy life. Food insecure households aren't necessarily food insecure all the time. It may reflect the need for families to make trade-offs for important needs such as transportation or medical bills in order to purchase nutritious food or vice versa.[13]

This is precisely why public produce can help eliminate hunger. As Pollan correctly surmised, foraging for entire meals is not feasible on a regular basis. But it doesn't have to be. Public produce isn't about doing away with Big Ag, supermarkets, or even farmers' markets. It's about increasing access to fresh, nutritious food in your community, so that if you find yourself—on occasion— pinched for time or money, you can still feed yourself and your family. No one should go hungry. Public produce can help ensure no one ever will.

The ability to forage in the city also brings benefits to those for whom hunger is not a problem, and who have the financial where-withal to not only eat well, but dine out often. Restaurateurs need regular access to high-quality, low-cost food to remain competitive. It matters little if the restaurant is a tony venue in the heart of downtown, or a mom-and-pop on the commercial strip; profit margins in the restaurant business are tight. The ability to offer diners the highest-quality food while controlling costs and maintaining profits is not easy. Supermarkets offer low-cost ingredients, but generally of lower quality. Farmers' markets have high-quality produce, but at a premium. A system of public produce could provide mutual benefit for the restaurateur and diner by ensuring a supply of low-cost, high-quality food.

Public produce also has value beyond a low purchase price. Many restaurateurs insist on locally grown food. Indeed, it is the use of local ingredients that often distinguishes fine eating establishments from mediocre ones. Ambiance and culinary talents may not be sufficient in today's competitive restaurant market. It is the provenance of the food that is becoming increasingly important, and many patrons now judge quality based on the distance food has traveled from the field to their plate. Being able to forage in the city for fresh, quality ingredients sates the discriminating diner's appetite for locally grown food.

Public produce can create symbiosis between restaurateur, forager, and city government. At the core of our most vibrant and convivial downtowns and urban neighborhoods are restaurants, cafés, and other eating establishments. A popular economic development strategy is to seed urban places with diverse places of food consumption. Even developers of today's suburban shopping centers are seeking eateries—not department stores—to anchor their developments. Eateries provide entertainment throughout the day and well into the evening, and attract repeat customers. They add to the culture and nightlife of the city, and the best neighborhoods are imbued with generous helpings of them. It is only natural for cities to want to guarantee the financial success of eateries, and if locally grown food is becoming a requisite for today's menus, then it certainly behooves the city to ensure such food is within city limits at low cost.

I remember vividly an excellent *pastificio* in Berkeley's "Gourmet Ghetto" that went to what many would consider extraordinary lengths to secure high-quality, locally sourced produce at a reduced cost. An artfully hand-drawn sign prominently displayed in the storefront read, "Wanted: Meyer Lemons for Trade or Purchase." As Meyer lemon trees are fairly common in residential gardens throughout the Bay Area, I went inside to inquire a bit more about the offer. The counter person informed me the pastificio uses Meyer lemons in a variety of recipes, such as the specialty pastas and baked goods they produce. Many chefs and gourmands prefer this lemon variety for its distinctively sweet, orange-lemony flavor. Because of demand, Meyer lemons are difficult to obtain in quantity from local grocery stores, and those that do carry them charge a premium.

"If a person comes in off the street with a box of Meyer lemons, you would buy them?" I asked.

"Yes," the woman at the counter replied. "If the person wants cash, we pay a dollar per pound. Or we are happy to offer baked goods or other menu items in exchange for the lemons."

I immediately realized there could be mutual benefit with this particular offer, between the restaurant and a forager less fortunate. I was suspicious, however, believing that what the owners may have unconsciously envisioned when they posted the sign was a well-to-do, middle-aged woman waltzing in with a box of Meyer lemons from her backyard garden.

Thinking there may be an opportunity here for those hit hardest financially, I asked the young lady, "What if a disheveled street person came in with a box of lemons? Would you still buy them or offer food in exchange?"

"Not necessarily . . ."

"Why?" I interrupted. "Are the lemons somehow unfit for human consumption simply because they have been handled by a street person?!"

"No, it's not that," she answered. "They can't be any lemons. They have to be *Meyer* lemons."

Obviously this offer is unique, but I held a new appreciation for Meyer lemons as the most prized of citrus fruit. As I left, I couldn't help but think that if only there were Meyer lemons to forage from the urban environment, those struggling to make ends meet could make a modest commission or enjoy delicious, freshly prepared

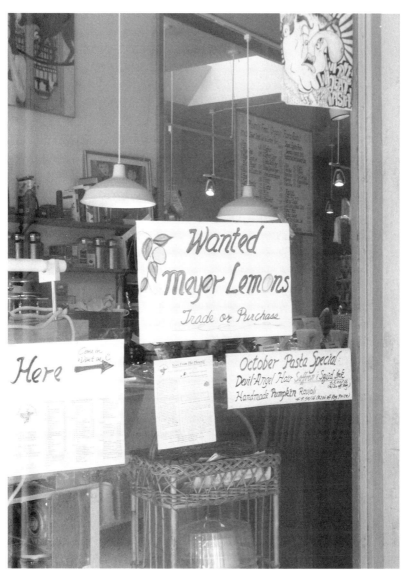

Meyer lemons—a favorite of gourmet cooks—command a premium price and are difficult to obtain in quantity. This Berkeley, California, pastificio offers to purchase neighborhood Meyer lemons at a modest price or barter for baked goods, in order to reduce overhead costs.

food in the warm and cozy atmosphere of this Italian bakery. This was certainly no soup kitchen.

As good as the pasta and baked goods were from this eatery, rents and other overhead costs proved too high, and the pastificio closed its storefront. The sign asking for Meyer lemons, though I had not recognized it at the time, was a public plea for help. I do not know to what extent a regular supply of low-cost Meyer lemons could have altered the fate of the pastificio, but I like to think that any opportunity to cut overhead costs could have saved this restaurant, or at least increased its longevity. As it is, the community lost a beloved business.

Not long after the pastificio shut its doors, I came across two healthy Meyer lemon shrubs growing in the public right-of-way between the sidewalk and the street, not more than three blocks from where the pastificio once operated. Remembering their unique cash- or barter-offer, and thinking of the mutual benefit that could exist between restaurateur and forager, I looked at these lemons in an entirely different light. For some, those yellow fruits are as good as gold.

Some restaurateurs forage not out of financial necessity, but out of principle. Chez Panisse, the internationally acclaimed restaurant and shining star of Berkeley's Gourmet Ghetto, is certainly in no danger of closing its doors anytime soon. Its popularity and success have sustained it for four decades, owing to the culinary talents and slow-food philosophy of Alice Waters and her talented staff. Serving the freshest locally sourced food is a large reason for the restaurant's success, and has helped grow Berkeley's reputation as one of the greatest foodie centers in the country.

Staff at Chez Panisse regularly forage for ingredients for their daily menu items. Many of the tarts, pies, and pastries prepared by the restaurant are filled with fruit foraged from various neighborhoods—fruit that is either difficult to source even from farmers' markets, or particularly expensive. According to Stacie Pierce, the pastry chef at Chez Panisse, as much as 30 percent of the fruit used for pastries is foraged. Meyer lemons, blood oranges, huckleberries, kiwi fruit, bitter almonds, black walnuts, persimmons, passion fruits, kumquats, pears, apples, blackberries, mulberries, and raspberries are a few of the foraged fruits that find their way into Stacie's pastries. Some of the items are brought in by locals. Stacie recalls a woman who was hiking in Santa Cruz, and showed up at the restaurant's door one day with a basket of huckleberries. Others arrive with foraged mushrooms from the Berkeley hills, like the prized, golden-colored chanterelles. What has always distinguished Chez Panisse from other restaurants is its flexibility—the ability to change the menu based on what is not only available but at its freshest and most flavorful. "If you have found something truly amazing," Stacie says, "you don't have to ask if we can use it. We *will* work it into the menu."[14] Though the restaurant readily accepts foraged food from locals, staff prefers to forage for food themselves. These culinary artists have developed the talent to recognize when food is at its peak of flavor. Sometimes, the restaurant has to turn away foraged food brought in from neighbors, simply because it does not meet the staff's high standards for quality. But through rejection, the forager becomes better educated on food and food quality and, over time, develops an appreciation and keen sense of food usually mastered only by talented chefs.

While even restaurateurs and patrons of critically acclaimed restaurants can benefit from food foraged within their urban surrounds, their sustenance is more psychological than physical. Locally sourced produce gives diners satisfaction largely based on environmental principles, beliefs toward improved health, or notions of improved flavor. Some in this country have the luxury of choosing what, when, and how often they eat and where their food comes from. Others do not possess such luxuries. Opportunities to glean and forage for food offer society's less fortunate—those with limited options in life—a choice. While we are starting to see a growing number of middle-class and well-to-do folks benefit from gleaning and foraging in the city, the biggest benefactors will always be the most financially challenged.

Back in Berkeley, a man sits idly near a mature redwood tree in Ohlone Park. Richard is homeless, and sleeps every night under the relative protection of the tree's canopy. His behavior and demeanor are not what we typically associate with homeless people. Richard is well-spoken, congenial, and, all things considered, well dressed. He doesn't appear to suffer from any psychological or substance-abuse problems, and there are never any empty beer cans or liquor bottles near the area where he sleeps. Every morning, after Richard awakes and stretches, he stuffs his bedroll in a backpack, along with a few modest belongings, and heads downtown in search of food and social contact.

Richard, like many homeless people, is a middle-aged person with limited education, few skills, and no family. Nevertheless, he is articulate, well mannered, and wise in ways that well-heeled college graduates may never be. I ask Richard if he would find it desirable if fruit trees were planted in the park. "I think it would be," he replies. "There are many days I wish there was just a peach tree around here."

I find it interesting that it is not necessarily "things" that people with little in the world crave, but experiences. For Richard, it wasn't just any fruit he desired in the park, but specifically a peach. It has been a long time since Richard tasted a peach, and it became evident that he wasn't just craving food for simple sustenance, but the experience it yielded. A peach's flavor, aroma, and juiciness provided fond memories for Richard, memories of when he was younger— memories of when he was in a better, more stable situation in life.

We cannot underestimate the value of enriched experiences in our daily lives (recall Solomon's essay, "Peaches"). Picking fruit from a tree is more enriching than buying it from the supermarket—both spiritually and financially. For Richard, the ability to pluck a peach off a tree is more than convenient sustenance. It is the opportunity to return to some semblance of self-sufficiency, by not having to rely entirely on handouts from others, while recapturing an innocent joy of youth that has value for Richard. He now worries he may never taste a peach again, because of his particular economic station. But Richard's real problem isn't his lack of money. Rather, it is the modern ways that food is produced in this country and made available to people in the city. A person's depleted finances should not prohibit him from eating a fresh peach.

Richard mentioned that the bulk of his time each day is spent searching for food. It was then that I realized, for some, time is just as important as money for those deepest in debt. Searching in trash bins or begging for money to buy meals is very time-consuming, and often yields food that is at best palatable, and at worst, harmful. Many homeless, like Richard, could have more time to seek employment or education if they did not have to spend so much time in search of food. Having fresh produce readily available and accessible provides not only more healthful sustenance, but freedom and time to pursue other necessities in life.

I talk to Richard more about the idea of planting a variety of food-bearing plants in public spaces throughout the city. He points to the community garden in the park, "Well they have a vegetable garden over there. The only problem is that nobody like me can get in." Richard has an interesting point. The posted sign reads, "Ohlone Community Garden." Along the bottom of the sign are hastily painted letters, "*No Entrar.*" The garden, surrounded by a five-foot-tall chain-link fence, has only one access point. This point of entry is secured with a padlock and, for extra protection, a combination lock. Obviously, food here is highly valuable, and some members of the community are doing their best to keep other members of the public out of community plots on public land. What is most disconcerting is the racial bias to the message. One wonders whether there is proof that Hispanics are responsible for stealing the produce, or is it just an assumption?

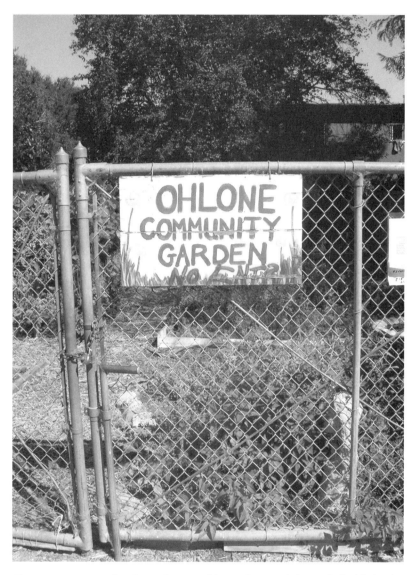

This community garden, located in a public park in Berkeley, is locked behind a chain-link fence with a padlock and, for added security, a combination lock. Most disturbing is the racially biased directive, "No Entrar."

It is in these instances when one realizes that perhaps community gardens are a misnomer. Though they may be located on public land, the typical community garden only benefits a few individuals—individuals who sometimes go to great lengths to keep the "community" out of their community gardens. Public produce should benefit all by providing for all, where food grown on public land is not locked behind fences, but is freely accessible and available to everyone. One of the greatest shortcomings—and ironies —of traditional community gardens is their personal, privatized nature. The people who typically benefit from community gardens are only those individuals who put down a monetary deposit for a plot; pay for their own plants, fertilizer, and compost; and take the time to sow, tend, and harvest the gardens. It is understandable why most would choose not to share food with others who do nothing to help purchase, plant, or maintain the garden, and many will argue this is only fair, and how it should be. America is not a socialist country, after all. But America has a growing population of have-nots, and the strength of this country is directly tied to the health and wealth of all our citizens. Surely, individuals should have the freedom to garden, and the right to keep everything they sow and reap for themselves. But we must also recognize that *The Little Red Hen* ethos of community gardening does little to benefit the greater community.

It is important to point out other limitations, or at least misconceptions, of traditional community gardens, because they are often regarded as the ultimate safety net for many of our food problems. In his more than thirty-five years of urban agriculture experience and community food service, author Mark Winne admits that our often idealistic claims of self-reliance through community gardening "come precariously close to self-righteous pontificating." Winne explains that "having witnessed the many sincere but ultimately failed attempts to transform dirt, water, and seed into food, I tend to look somewhat askance at those who suggest that more of us, if not all of us, and especially the poor, should 'grow their own.'"[15]

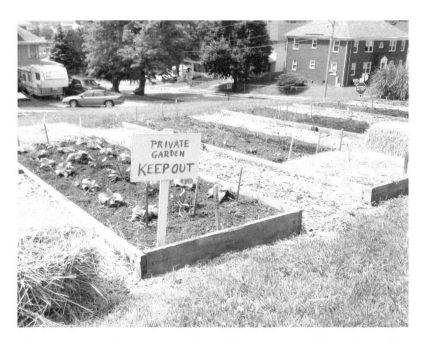

The privatization of community garden produce is sometimes blatantly—and, at times, ridiculously—obvious. The fact that the public pilfers the veggies underscores the need for opportunities to forage.

Winne's point is that many fail to recognize the effort, knowledge, and resources that are necessary to grow food. There will always be citizens who lack the skills to grow fresh produce (children, for example), the time (because they work two jobs to make ends meet, attend night school, or are single parents), the strength and dexterity (many elderly and disabled), or the financial resources to purchase seed, soil, and tools (the impoverished). For these individuals and others, there should be opportunities to gather food.

Another shortcoming with traditional community gardens is that they allow municipal government to appease a persistent citizen group without much effort on the government's part. In many communities, the local officials do little more than give permission to a group to plant vegetables on city-owned land—often on vacant lots the city has acquired that nobody wants anyway. Sure, the municipality might pay the water bill, and perhaps offer compost, but these products are not paid for collectively by the taxpayers; they are often paid from the fees that municipalities levy against citizens wishing to garden. Some municipalities do not even want that level of involvement, which often necessitates a third, not-for-profit party, like a *Friends of the* (insert name here) *Community Garden*. These groups are responsible for securing funding, managing the supplies, paying the water bill, policing, and other efforts, with little to no assistance from the municipality. In short, many forms of community gardening represent a very hands-off approach to urban agriculture for the municipality. What is necessary, I am arguing, is for municipalities to adopt a more proactive, hands-on policy.

Community gardens are undoubtedly beneficial to cities, and are currently the largest component of urban agriculture today. There is no disputing the good that is intended with community gardens, and land should be set aside for more of them. At the heart of any successful urban agriculture endeavor, now and in the future, are community gardens. These will most likely supply the greatest diversity of produce, but such diversity can require the most labor. However, community gardens alone cannot feed an entire community, as their semiprivate nature eliminates any possibility for people (other than those tending the plots) to forage. A balance needs to be struck between community gardens on public land (maintained as if they were private), and *true* public produce, meaning food available to all. Public food gardens, spearheaded and managed by public officials, like the fruit orchards in Calgary and the City Hall vegetables in Provo, will have to supplement conventional citizen-driven community gardens. The role of city government that endorses the concept of true public produce is to manage and tend public gardens with available municipal resources and talent, or else hire the skilled and the learned to ensure the health and well-being of the plants, which will ensure the health and well-being of the community.

Some argue that providing access to healthy, low-cost food is not the role of city government. As long as city planners and elected officials strive to create programs to reduce social inequity, and increase the quality of life for their citizens, I contend it is. For the same reasons that city governments provide clean drinking water, protection from crime and catastrophe, shelters and low-income housing programs, sewage treatment, garbage collection, fallen-tree disposal, and pothole-free streets, access to healthy, low-cost food helps ensure the health, safety, and welfare of the city's citizens. The surest manner to provide nutritious, affordable food for those citizens is to create opportunities to glean and forage in the city.

Poverty is likely intractable, but hunger does not have to be. Public officials need to recognize hunger's pervasiveness across the country, and fight to eliminate it. Programs and policies need to be crafted and resources set aside to ensure that all of life's basic necessities are met: health care, shelter, clothing, as well as food. Gleaning and foraging for fresh produce can directly meet people's needs for food, and may indirectly help them meet the other three life necessities. Eating healthier can obviously reduce the number of illnesses and subsequent doctor visits attributable to poor diet, and if food can be had for little to no cost, enough money may be spared to help purchase clothing, or even make rent. Some individuals, to be certain, are beyond the financial means to acquire additional clothing or shelter, even if there were an extensive system of public produce. But for many single-parent families, elderly, and working poor, a fine line is walked between solvency and ruin, and every penny helps.

Chapter 5

Maintenance and Aesthetics

W HO IS GOING TO TAKE CARE OF IT?" This is the perennial question every time food in public space is proposed. Though the question is certainly valid, it is usually asked rhetorically.

Municipal officials are quick to point out that edibles are messy and difficult to maintain. Not only that, but vegetable and fruit gardens are untidy, scruffy landscapes; wholly inappropriate for our manicured public settings. Peaches in a public plaza will just make a squishy mess on the pavement. And those vine-ripened, baseball-sized tomatoes just beg to be thrown at windows, cars, and passersby![1]

While some types of fruit and nut trees provide basis for these concerns, and only then in certain public settings (and only then if nobody harvests the food before it drops), there is a lot of hypocrisy over edibles being inappropriate plants for the urban environment. Public officials and those caring for and maintaining our landscaped grounds need to take a more critical—and objective—look at the varieties of plants commonly planted in our parks and plazas. Once we look with a keen eye toward the nature in our cities, it becomes evident that the plants commonly found in our public spaces are just as messy as many of our familiar food-bearing plants—sometimes more so.

For example, you might argue that apple trees are too messy for public spaces. Ornamental flowering plums, on the other hand, are widely considered a fantastic addition to any urban landscape, and are frequently planted in cities throughout the country because they are one of the few trees that bloom in winter. Some cultivars even have purple leaves, making them highly desirable because of their unusual foliage. Flowering plums do produce fruit, though it has little edible value. (The fruit is only about one inch in diameter with a largish stony pit.) While many praise the unique foliage color of some varieties, and the magnificent beauty of the delicate blossoms, the fruit drop can be extremely messy, as the flesh and juice from these little plums are quite effective at staining not only pavement, but the hoods of cars as well.

The ornamental flowering cherry, like its cousin the flowering plum, is also prized in the urban landscape. Yet it, too, produces an abundance of small, inedible fruit, which poses both a maintenance burden and liability risk during fruit drop. But cherry blossoms take our breath away, and such beauty ensures that these trees will remain prized in the urban landscape.

Strawberry tree is a popular small tree in western landscapes, admired not for its flowers, but its gorgeous clusters of multicolored fruit. Scores of little orange, red, and yellow drupes burst from leathery, dark green leaves, like sun-splashed confetti. Though the fruit can be made into jellies, it is generally considered too bland and mealy to be palatable. These visually striking fruits are soft and squishy, turning light-colored concrete into a darkened and stained eyesore.

Victorian box is a beloved urban street tree, widely used in cities with temperate climates. The thousands of orange berries that each tree produces, though visually stunning, provide a sticky mess, frustrating both pedestrians and motorists unlucky enough to park their cars under the tree during fruit drop. Cotoneaster and pyracantha (firethorn) are favorites among landscape architects because of their profusion of brightly colored red and orange berries. But these berries provide only eye candy, as they are unpalatable to humans; and they, too, make quite a mess.

Yellow pine pollen coats everything within a breeze's reach, and acacias not only aggravate allergies, but also require sidewalk cleanup during flower drop. Bottlebrush and jacaranda drop flowers with sticky nectar. Leaf litter is a problem with Chinese elm, redwoods, pines, and cedars. Sweetgum and red horsechestnut —popular street trees in the South and Mid-Atlantic, prized respectively for their brilliant fall color and spring blossoms—drop dozens of hard, one-inch-diameter seed capsules to the sidewalk and street. These capsules present a safety hazard and potential liability, as people could slip or roll their ankles on the round pods.

The fantastic aesthetics of our most prized landscape plants makes it easy for us to forget that they produce an abundance of leaf litter, drip with sticky nectar, and drop unpalatable fruit by the bunches. Persimmon, fig, Asian pear, lemon, banana, orange, pomegranate, almond, and scores of other food-bearing plants possess equal pizzazz, in addition to their delicious and nutritious fruit. Passion vine, for instance, is an excellent alternative to trumpet vine, offering a more exotic-looking flower and wonderfully aromatic fruit.[2] Grapevines trained to ramble over pergolas and along white picket fences provide both beauty and sustenance. They make wonderful substitutes for wisteria—a plant often used for its fragrance and visual display of long, drooping clusters of flowers. Instead of clusters of flowers, think clusters of berries; one titillates our sense of smell, the other our sense of taste.

Wild strawberry and creeping thyme are both vigorous, low-maintenance groundcovers. Kale, cabbage, radicchio, and chard are tidy, no-mess additions to any perennial bed. Ornamental

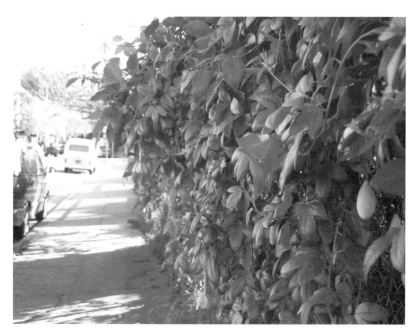

Passion vine provides an aesthetically pleasing—and exotically edible—screen to an otherwise unfriendly chain-link fence. The particular variety shown here, banana passion fruit (Passiflora mollisima), can be grown in temperate climates, making it more useful in many parts of the country than its subtropical cousin, purple passion fruit (Passiflora edulis).

grasses, such as purple fountain grass and switchgrass, have become quite popular in landscapes, providing a lacy, feathery accent that hints at wildness. These grasses are often praised by environmentalists because of their drought tolerance. Fennel can provide a similarly lacy, wild look, and is every bit as drought tolerant as ornamental grasses. Rosemary, marjoram, and oregano are about as maintenance-free as plants get, providing drought-tolerant alternatives that are handsome, fragrant, and edible.

There are also degrees of messiness. What is worse, a conifer that dribbles sticky sap and drops needles throughout the year, or a deciduous tree that releases its leaves all at once? Is an apple tree that drops fruit once a year more of a maintenance headache than a silver

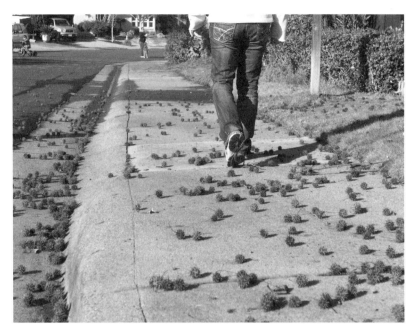

Sweet gums (Liquidambar styraciflua) *are prized street trees across much of the United States. The scores of hard, round seed pods dropped from each tree arguably provide as much risk to pedestrians as fallen fruit and nuts.*

maple that heaves and breaks sidewalks at maturity? These questions are difficult to answer definitively. The real issue, rather, is that almost all trees and shrubs are messy, and fallen fruit, branches, wet leaves, and sticky flowers—regardless of whether the plant is ornamental or edible—require cleanup and pose some aesthetic affront.

The point is, we shouldn't indiscriminately dismiss food-bearing plants in public landscapes because of perceptions that they are ugly and labor intensive. Plants provide a greater good than simple aesthetics. For municipalities that accept a philosophy that food security is one of those greater goods, attention should turn to strategies that can feed hungry citizens without placing an undue burden on maintenance staff.

Fortunately, a few cities in the United States and Canada have figured out how to include food in their public places economically and handsomely, by choosing certain plants over others, mixing edibles with ornamentals, utilizing existing maintenance staff and methods, and properly gauging community demand for fresh, local produce.

The management plan for edibles—as with ornamentals—is bifurcated. The first branch of maintenance is the ongoing care of the plant: the watering and weeding, pruning and mulching, fertilizing and pest control. The second branch is cleanup. For ornamentals, this means gathering the fallen leaves, flowers, and fruit and disposing of the litter. For edibles, it means harvesting the fruit *before* it falls.

Let's begin with the second fork of managing food in the landscape, since that gives municipal officials the most anxiety. How to harvest fruit, nuts, and vegetables without placing physical and financial burden on the municipality? If you look at food harvesting as an opportunity rather than a liability, there is great potential to turn maintenance headaches into moneymakers. Which is exactly what the University of California at Davis discovered, offering a lucrative lesson to every municipality.

Olive trees—close to 1,500 of them—line walkways, bike paths, and other public spaces on the Davis campus, creating not only a maintenance nightmare for the grounds crew, but a real liability for the school as well. Navigating through the squished fruits and stony pits requires considerable caution. It is manageable for pedestrians, but in this bicycling community, fallen fruit can prove treacherous to those on two wheels. In 2004, sixty thousand dollars was spent in legal fees for bicycle accidents related to olive drop. This was in addition to the annual cost of another sixty thousand dollars just to clean up and dispose of the olives.

It was a never-ending nightmare for Sal Genito, director of the university's Buildings and Grounds Division. One day, after he was called to the site of a particularly bad bicycle accident, he had an epiphany. Genito was surveying the scene of the accident alongside

Russell Boulevard, an area where hundreds of olive trees line the space between the bike path and the street. Smashed olives were everywhere, creating an extremely slick surface that was made even more treacherous with light rain. As Genito pondered solutions to this incredible mess, an inescapable aroma hit his nose: olive oil! So he bought a small press, picked some fresh olives, and churned out a fragrant and delicious green-hued liquid—and UC Davis Olive Oil was branded.

In the fall of 2004, the first olive-oil vintage of UC Davis, 80 gallons of artisan extra-virgin olive oil was pressed and bottled. It was an immediate hit with consumers, and production has increased substantially since. The 2006 vintage yielded almost 450 gallons, and sold out in just four months. The 2007 vintage produced close to 800 gallons of oil (which, by the way, comes in three distinct blends, depending on the varieties of olives used). At twelve to fifteen dollars per 250-milliliter bottle, the financial returns are staggering. The 2007 vintage generated close to eighty thousand dollars in profit, which helped create the UC Davis Olive Center, an education and research facility devoted to the production of olives and olive oil. Today, the Olive Center creates not only some of the finest olive oil this side of the Mediterranean, but an assortment of artisan olive products, like luxurious soaps, lotions, and balms. A simple yet ingenious idea that sprouted from a hazardous nuisance, UC Davis's olive-oil program not only generates enough revenue to cover maintenance and liability costs of fruit drop on public space, but has an entire research division that fosters widespread understanding and appreciation of this gustatory delight.[3]

Here is what is bearing out across the country: folks are growing wary of distant food conglomerates and instead favor community-produced foods. Ironically, those who can afford to will typically pay more for food grown locally. What this means is local food has immense value. UC Davis's olive oil and the City of Chicago's honey are just two examples of innovative strategies that turn

maintenance crews into moneymakers by sating our hunger for locally produced food. Similar strategies merit consideration; not only
for fresh produce, but for the various dried fruits and vegetables,
preserves, jams, jellies, nut and seed butters, oils, relishes, and other
value-added foodstuffs that could be produced by the municipality
and sold back to the community. Food is a resource with great entrepreneurial value. Within an effort to manage fruit drop and to offset
maintenance costs, there are opportunities to provide local folk with
local food, and receive handsome remuneration for the effort.

The prospect of turning fruit trees into money trees is certainly
provocative. But most bureaucrats don't fancy themselves entrepreneurs, and the imperative to earn a profit seldom drives maintenance goals. For public officials like Callie Le'au Cartright, finding
a simple, cost-neutral solution to fallen fruit has value enough.

Callie is the parks supervisor for the City of Des Moines, and the
overseer of the municipality's community garden program. As she
or any community garden coordinator will tell you, folks are gung
ho to garden come April, but by August that gumption—along
with the tomatoes, basil, and beans—wilts in the summer sun. Not
only does precious, garden fresh food go to waste, but somebody
has to tidy the unkempt beds. In Des Moines that somebody is Callie and her crew, adding burden to an already overtaxed staff.

But there was a more vexing problem than overgrown garden
plots littered with forgotten food. Callie mentioned the interest in
community gardening has grown substantially in Des Moines. Yet
Des Moines, like cities across the country, is seeing a decline in
food security. Folks who need fresh fruits and vegetables the most
have the poorest access to produce. It isn't the hungry who are
tending those community garden plots.

Callie saw a solution. She formed what she calls a food rescue
committee. This committee comprises volunteers who rove the
city's hundreds of community garden beds, plucking neglected
fruits and veggies before they molder. The group then distributes

the bounty of fresh produce to local food pantries, curtailing food waste while ensuring the city's hungry eat well. This committee provides another win-win for the community: not only does locally grown, fresh produce get to those who need it most, but harvesting neglected food keeps Callie's community gardens neat and tidy.

Of course, not all strategies to eliminate food waste need to be entrepreneurial or innovative. The simplest solution to manage fallen fruit could prove to be just as effective. A sign, artfully written and conspicuously placed, encouraging folks to harvest ripe produce may be all that is needed to curtail neglect. What I have witnessed in my many years of managing and promoting public produce is that people are reluctant to harvest public edibles because they perceive them as private. "Surely these ripe plums aren't meant for me," we think.

Our reluctance to pluck from the public fruit tree is logical. After all, we are not accustomed to seeing food growing right before us in our urban surrounds, free for the picking. This change in context—from one where we give somebody money for food to one where it is offered free of charge—will take some getting used to. Until then, a simple message of encouragement can help ease our hesitancy.

The most efficient way to ensure little to zero waste is to match the food supply with consumer demand. In other words, maintenance can be minimized when we effectively estimate what I call the "carrying capacity" of public produce. The question is not how many plum trees can you plant in a park. Rather, the question is how many plums *should* you plant?

Municipalities interested in edible landscapes need to consider the number of people passing by each and every public space, and whether those people are likely to consume the quantity and type of food offered. For example, you could line a suburban street with persimmon trees spaced forty feet apart. But this is bad practice. Why? Because all those trees would yield an overabundance of fruit for the relative paucity of residents in the typical low-density

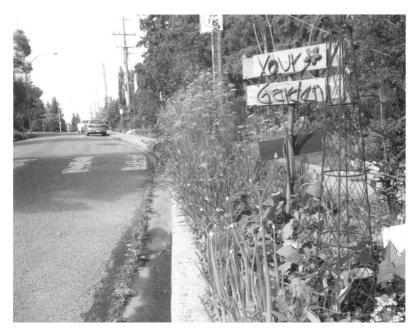

A whimsical sign in Edmonton, Alberta, reminds passersby that sidewalk produce is public produce. (Courtesy of Jennifer Cockrall-King)

subdivision. And Americans have yet to develop a fondness for persimmon. The result would be a lot of unwanted fruit.

Conversely, a single peach tree in the center of a bustling campus quad may not yield enough fruit for the thousands of hungry, cash-strapped college students. Matching expected crop yields to numbers of people likely to harvest the produce is paramount in reducing urban agricultural surplus.

The importance of proper carrying capacity became evident while I was living in Berkeley. What caught me by surprise was the general lack of fruit on the ground from the many neighborhood fruit trees. Many of Berkeley's neighborhoods are densely populated, and even along quieter streets, scores of people pass by on foot or bicycle daily.

On Grant Street, for example, just a few blocks northwest of downtown, a fifteen-foot-tall navel orange tree thrives in the

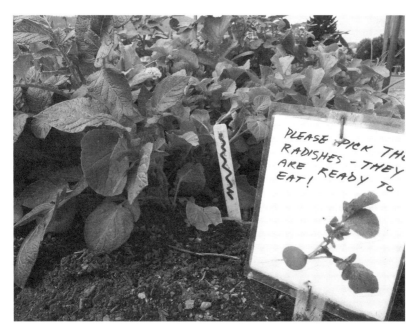

Handwritten signs urge passersby to pick what's ripe in Kamloops, British Columbia. (Courtesy of Elaine Sedgman)

narrow planting bed wedged between the sidewalk and curb. In the middle of February, dozens of good-sized fruit were ripe and ready to pick. The only problem was they were out of reach. And only a couple of oranges lay on the ground. Most of the ripe fruit that would ordinarily be within an arm's reach had already been harvested, providing winter treats for the neighborhood.

On Channing Street, a few blocks south of that orange tree, another fruit tree thrives in the skinny bit of landscape between the street and sidewalk. This one is a fig tree, and when the fruit is ripe, few are ever found on the ground. Figs are prized fruit, after all, similar to oranges, and I suspect this is partially why there is little waste.

One day, as I was admiring all the ripe figs, the homeowner who cared for the tree emerged from his house. "Help yourself," he kindly offered. "They didn't do so well this year, but they're still okay, and we can't eat them all anyway."

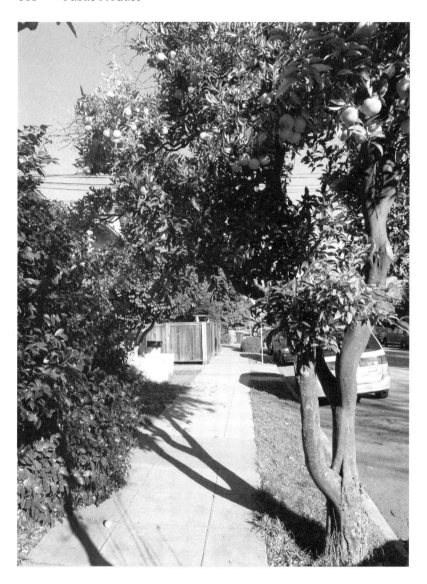

I asked him when he planted the tree. "Five years ago," he responded.

"Have any of the neighbors or city people ever complained about fruit drop, or mess during that time?"

"No, not at all," he said. "There's really not that much that falls

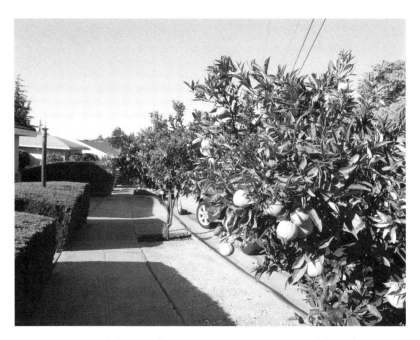

Orange trees in Berkeley, California. The remarkable absence of fallen fruit proves that public produce is prized in some communities.

to the ground. We pick some, but I think other people occasionally pick the fruit as well. Actually, the leaves make more of a mess during the winter when they all fall off, but nobody complains about that either."

Three blocks west of downtown, between the orange tree on Grant Street and the fig tree on Channing, an apple tree grows in Ohlone Park. Typical of most urban settings, this neighborhood park attracts a diversity of citizens. Dog walkers, teenagers, stroller-pushing parents, idle elderly, and a few homeless congregate here daily. In November, when the apples are ripe, few fruits can be found littering the grass below. The canopy of the tree still houses scores of hanging fruit, but most are outside of a normal person's reach. But soon, even the fruit high up in the tree will disappear. Like the orange and fig trees observed in the neighborhood, this tree is feeding folks.

These three fruit trees demonstrate proper carrying capacity for this Berkeley neighborhood. How? Because few fruits ever litter the sidewalks below. That which is produced is picked and eaten. Indeed, the lack of fruits on the ground may warrant *more* fruit trees planted in Berkeley's public spaces.

Many factors must be weighed when determining the proper carrying capacity of public space. First is estimating the degree to which locals desire public fruits and vegetables. In Berkeley, that desire is extremely high. Berkeley has a strong food culture, and citizens there prize fresh, locally grown produce. This insatiable desire, along with the sheer number of people who pass by the fruit trees in this high-density neighborhood, guarantees little waste.

Visibility is also important in managing food litter: Where food is planted within a particular space is just as important as how much food is produced. If edibles are planted in a back corner of a seldom-used park, expect lots of waste. Food should be prominently displayed in the landscape, reminding people of their food choices, and inviting them to harvest. The three trees in that Berkeley neighborhood are all in plain sight. It is obvious to anyone passing by that the fruit is in public space, accessible from a sidewalk and thus available to all, regardless of who tends them.

Managing food drop is arguably the most worrisome issue with regard to edibles, but it is an issue that generally needs attention only once each year. Keeping edible landscapes healthy and thriving year-round can be more perplexing to maintenance crews. It involves continual irrigation, mulching, weeding, pruning, and pest management. Public officials will perennially argue there is simply no budget to hire gardeners to maintain a network of public produce. Those arguments seem particularly valid with lean municipal budgets. But planting food does not necessitate hiring additional maintenance staff. Instead, municipalities can tap the skills of their existing workers within a broad range of government departments.

One department especially suited for the maintenance of public produce is parks and recreation. This department employs skilled laborers to maintain a city's myriad green spaces. Sure, some seasonal hires may know little beyond mowing lawns, blowing leaves, and pruning shrubs into sumptuous gumballs. But many others also know how to plant and stake trees, transplant shrubs, mulch planting beds, weed, deadhead, prune, and fertilize the city's ornamental landscapes. These skills are exactly what are necessary to grow edibles. In other words, public grounds are already being maintained with skilled labor, so it is not a matter of hiring new staff, or even retraining existing staff. It is more a matter of redefining how workers are currently maintaining public spaces.

The forestry department is another division well suited to the maintenance of public produce. Forestry staff are already tasked with the management of a city's urban trees. And these departments are typically headed by certified arborists—professionals who understand the intimate needs of all sorts of woody plants, ornamental as well as edible.

Take Chris Johnson, for example, the city arborist for Davenport, Iowa. Johnson is a public servant and an entrepreneur. And he is blazing new trails in urban forestry.

One initiative Johnson is pioneering is urban wood utilization, an environmentally friendly manner of producing building materials from storm-damaged and felled trees. He and his forestry crew mill lumber from the removed trees, and then sell that lumber back to the community. Eco-conscious woodworkers in Davenport now have a sustainable source of building materials for fences, tool sheds, and vegetable beds. Johnson and his crew also build Leopold benches from the lumber, and sell those at the farmers' market and city auctions. The money generated from selling the benches and raw lumber is funneled back into Davenport's General Fund, the same fund used to pay Johnson and his crew's salary.

Johnson also does something that other municipal arborists wouldn't touch with a ten-foot stick: he plants fruit and nut trees to improve community access to fresh produce. Since 2012, Johnson has planted 100 pawpaw, apple, and pecan trees in parks throughout the city. He is tasked with managing all of the public trees anyway, so why shouldn't a few of these bear fruit for the community? In addition to the pruning, thinning, and other maintenance, Johnson and his forestry crew will also coordinate the harvest once these young trees bear fruit. During particularly bountiful years, when there could be more fruit than his small crew can handle, Johnson says he will enlist the help of the Quad Cities Food Hub, a regional food system advocacy group that connects local food producers to consumers. The Quad Cities Food Hub will disperse the pawpaws, apples, and pecans throughout the community, via the farmers' market and the local food bank. In other words, Quad citizens will have a bounty of fresh, locally grown food, and none will be wasted.

For smaller public produce gardens, maintenance doesn't have to be undertaken by skilled contractors and licensed professionals. The planners in Provo, for example, prove that all that is needed is a few folks with green thumbs and a passion for food justice.

The beauty of growing food in public space is that there is usually staff assigned to the upkeep of the landscape. The care of food-bearing plants can be done by those same employees who tend the rest of the plants. But there is one network of public space—and it is a big one—that generally does not have municipal staff dedicated to landscape maintenance: streets.

Maintaining public gardens on streets is tricky. For one, streets are the most extensive public setting in any city, reaching every home and every business. And municipalities place far more restrictions on what gets planted along city streets than in city parks. Which is somewhat ironic, since upkeep is often left entirely to homeowners and merchants.[4]

Even in the food-forward cities of Berkeley and San Francisco, fruit and nut trees are outlawed along streets. San Francisco and Berkeley's urban forestry divisions operate in much the same way as other municipalities with regard to tree planting in the public right-of-way. If you want to plant a street tree, you need to obtain a permit. The City of San Francisco and the City of Berkeley do not plant fruit trees of any kind in the public right-of-way along streets, and citizens wishing to plant a fruit tree in one of these strips will be denied a permit. Yet it happens anyway throughout these two local-food-crazed communities, and municipal staff look the other way. But city government should take a more proactive role than turning a blind eye to enforcement of an unpopular ordinance.

Richard Register, a notable environmental planner and urban theorist who has spent decades investigating and promoting the food production potential in cities, understands well the consternation city officials have about fruit trees as street trees:

Fruit and nut trees are illegal along the streets of most cities. This is because some owners fail to harvest or clean up under their fruit trees, thus creating an aesthetic offense in other people's eyes and a liability if someone were to step on a fruit and slip. Both objections are legitimate but could be reduced in two ways. First, establish a legal procedure for taking responsibility for the trees: either the city hires a roving orchard farmer (city employees presently trim ornamental street trees in any case), or the landowner who wants the trees accepts responsibility for upkeep, and for liability and penalty. In this same spirit, the food-tree lover could strategically plant trees with soft fruit (plums, peaches, and some pears) where they do not overhang sidewalks, while reserving nuts and harder fruit (apples and lemons) for the more public locations. Second—and this is a matter of degree— people should take responsibility for themselves. To slip and fall on a sidewalk because of a fruit should not yield a gigantic settlement for the unalert person—a small settlement based on shared responsibility would make sense. Perhaps people who can't trust their own awareness should insure themselves; laws certainly should encourage transfer of a good deal of responsibility back to the individual.[5]

Public officials' concern over fallen fruit and liability along our streets is certainly real and at times valid (recall the olive trees along the streets in Davis, California). And Register's strategies offer a couple of methods to help protect the municipality. His suggestion that landowners be required to maintain fruit trees is very easy to implement, since a variation of this strategy is already commonplace throughout much of the United States. The requirement to keep sidewalks free of fruit litter is no different than, say, snow removal. In communities throughout the Midwest and Northeast, it is the homeowner's responsibility to remove snow from city sidewalks. Homeowners who fail to comply will have the walk shoveled by their city, at the owner's expense. Homeowners aren't thrilled about shoveling sidewalks, but few object to this policy. That is because the policy seems logical and just; after all, we consider the sidewalk an extension of our front yard. Ensuring fruit doesn't accumulate on the sidewalk is no different from ensuring snow doesn't accumulate.

Register's suggestion that the city hire roving orchardists also makes good economic sense. Or maybe I should say "economic *cents*" since we are really talking pennies per pound of food here. Indeed, public officials will be surprised to learn just how cost-effective contracting with professional fruit harvesters can be. As Seattle's City Fruit discovered, professional harvesters are cheaper than volunteers.

Gail Savina has some pretty valuable insights gleaned from her years as executive director of City Fruit. When she founded the organization in 2008, City Fruit relied heavily on volunteers for harvests. This meant staff time recruiting, organizing, and training scores of people. And each year, the process would start over, as previous volunteers bowed out and new ones showed up.

The first harvests in 2009 and 2010 cost City Fruit more than $1.50 per pound of fruit. "Which isn't sustainable," Savina admitted. In 2011, City Fruit utilized fewer volunteers and paid professional harvesters to pick the bulk of the fruit. The result?

A whopping 33 percent reduction in costs. In 2013, using paid harvesters, an efficient database, and streamlined harvest procedures, City Fruit reported an *additional* 40 percent in cost savings from 2011. In five years, City Fruit cut harvesting costs from $1.50 to just $0.61 per pound of fruit. When you factor in the revenue from selling a portion of the produce to restaurants and canners and jelly makers, harvest costs are cut in half. Factor in further the donations and grants given to City Fruit for their benevolent work, and the organization is in the black. Which is great news for grass roots organizations—and municipalities—with less than shoe string budgets. Tons of community fruit is harvested, sparing mess and waste, and fed right back to the community. The net cost is nil, but the value priceless.

City Fruit does most of its harvesting in the verdant settings of residential neighborhoods, since that is where the food is. Most of the trees they harvest from are private property, sprouting from the front and back yards of homes. Even if you do happen upon a public fruit tree or vegetable patch (in a center street median or the landscape strip between the sidewalk and curb, for example) you will likely find yourself surrounded by homes and gardens. But what about the commercial districts in our cities? Might there be opportunities for public food outside our shops and storefronts, cafés and eateries? Extending public produce to commercial strips is a bit more challenging, since garden space along these bustling corridors is harder to come by. Here, government officials or the chamber of commerce may want to work with individual business owners to promote public edibles in the public right-of-way. But where to plant the food?

The City of Des Moines figured out a way to add garden space along the concreted streets of downtown through a unique beautification program. The premise of the program is simple: merchants supply planters outside their storefronts, and Parks staff supply the soil and plants. Voilà! Instant gardens. Parks employees even maintain the plants, though some merchants prefer to do so themselves. Because the intent of the program is street beautification, the bulk of the vegetation is purely ornamental. But Parks also uses plants that are not only handsome, but tasty as well, like chard, kale, and sweet potatoes.

The City of Kamloops, British Columbia, has a similar program. Historically, their downtown planters were filled with flowers. But a community activist bent on food justice recently challenged the City Council to plant vegetables in the containers. For the past few years, tomatoes, cilantro, basil, thyme, and parsley could be seen gracing Victoria Street, the busiest, most vibrant thoroughfare in the downtown. The herbs are especially popular among the many restaurateurs along the corridor. And the Councillors have wagered a friendly competition among themselves, by adopting planters and trying to outdo one another with their prolific produce displays. Such displays provide not only a source of pride for these city officials but convenient sustenance for the public. Not only that, but Kamloops and Des Moines prove that edibles are beautiful, and a welcome addition to an intensely urban setting.

Commercial areas provide another opportunity for easier management of edibles along the sidewalk. For municipalities intrigued with the idea of public-space agriculture, but that want no part in maintaining or harvesting the food, upkeep can be transferred to private developers. This strategy would place conditions upon commercial developments, like shopping centers and office parks. The semipublic spaces of these developments—namely, the landscaped plazas and courtyards between the buildings—are suitable locations for public produce. Though the land is privately owned, the public is freely allowed—and even encouraged—to access the property.

Placing conditions on commercial development is commonplace, and something municipal planners routinely do. The benefit of edibles grown on commercial land is that the grounds are already maintained by professional landscape contractors. A simple condition of development that could prove a win-win for the municipality

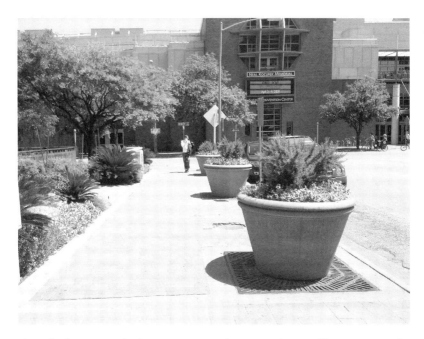

Giant herb pots outside this restaurant in downtown Austin add an engaging element to the streetscape and appear to require less maintenance than the street trees that once existed.

wanting to promote a system of public produce, but unable to maintain one, would be to require that 10 percent of all landscaped grounds be set aside for edibles with "permission to pass" granted to the public. The condition could further state that the edibles must remain healthy without the use of chemical fertilizers, herbicides, and pesticides, ensuring free, fresh, and organic produce.

Some developers don't need to be coerced into using edibles in their landscapes. Planners for the picturesque town of Nelson, British Columbia, recently started seeing fruit trees on the landscape plans for townhouse developments. The reasoning was logical: the developer felt that a few residents might like some garden fresh produce once in a while. While the City of Nelson never frowned upon edibles in private development, they hadn't encouraged their planting either.

But when planners began work on a long-range sustainability strategy for the community, it became obvious that food access and local food production are essential to meeting sustainable goals. The City of Nelson now has language in their Off-Street Parking and Landscape bylaws encouraging developers to construct edible landscapes.

Another compromise for municipalities wishing to support public agriculture but not wanting to manage it, is to ready public land for others to take over food production. This can easily be accommodated in the capital improvement programs of cities. Given the potential scale of some urban gardens, municipalities may be able to restore land to a productive, nutrient-rich medium far more economically than a small group of citizens can. This is especially true if the land has been developed or paved over, as with a parking lot. The amount of compost, machinery, and labor required to turn a sterile patch of dirt into fertile ground is too daunting for a few green thumbers. This is where government budgets and manpower can help.

After the ground is readied, it can then be turned over to the entrepreneurial farmer, neighborhood group, or not-for-profit organization for production and management of food. The one-time labor and capital expense shows commitment by the city for urban agriculture without placing ongoing maintenance demands on city staff.

The easiest—and most welcome—manner for a municipality to ready a site for food production is through a spigot. Regardless of who is responsible for the continual care and upkeep of our public landscapes, water is essential for healthy vegetation. Ironically, it is this simple necessity that is perennially missing from an otherwise fantastic farm or garden site. But the cost of running a water line to a vegetable patch is negligible; and if a community group is willing to garden and take on the maintenance of an otherwise neglected public space, everyone benefits, including the municipality. Which is why the lack of water to a street median in Seattle leaves Charlie Hoselton scratching his head.

Hoselton lives in Seattle's Queen Anne neighborhood along Gilman Drive West—a boulevard flanked with multistory condominiums and apartments. As with most densely populated urban neighborhoods, garden space in Queen Anne is scarce. Sure, there are a multitude of community gardens scattered throughout Seattle (one just a three-minute walk from where Hoselton lives). But in the Emerald City, community gardening is so popular that there are thousands on a wait list for a plot. The city just can't supply enough garden space to meet public demand.

But right outside Hoselton's door is a broad street median filled with vegetation. Well, weeds mainly, along with a few scrubby trees and invasive shrubs like Scotch broom. The dense vegetation was perfect for hiding all sorts of trash and illicit activity. Syringes and broken beer bottles were scattered amongst discarded tires, computer monitors, and an old television. These medians, once intended to add splendor to the street, had become a neighborhood eyesore.

Hoselton had an idea: he could transform one of the medians into a community garden, giving his neighbors a place to gather and garden, while reclaiming some of that lost splendor. He approached Seattle's Department of Transportation, promising to build and maintain the gardens himself with the help of his neighbors. Hoselton's team would off-haul all the debris, trim the overgrown trees, dig up the weeds, till the soil, and build the raised beds. It was an attractive offer for all parties, and Hoselton was given permission.

The median renovation has been a smashing success, and it really showcases what great community gardens can be. There are two dozen raised beds assigned to neighbors. Public fruit trees dot the median, giving anyone passing by access to garden fresh produce. A modest tool shed was placed in the middle of the site, while picnic tables and Adirondack chairs create a sort of front porch to the garden. To witness folks lounging and gardening in the middle of the street is a fantastically unique experience, something offered

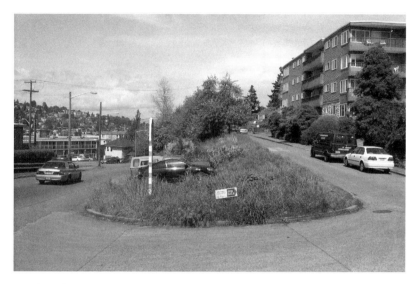

Weeds and overgrown vegetation plague the street medians on Gilman Drive West, Seattle.

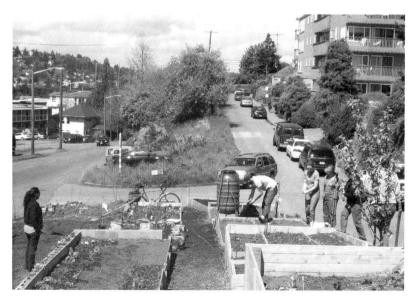

One of the medians now transformed into a community garden and gathering space.

only through great urban settings. The median has everything a city gardener could want, except one thing: water.

If you think it rains so much in Seattle there is no need for supplemental water in a garden, you haven't visited the city in the summer. Though most months the city is under a perpetual rain cloud, from July through August—prime gardening time—the city receives a scant two inches of precipitation, the same amount as Phoenix. Two weeks of hot, dry weather can ruin months of cultivation.

The Gilman Gardens have been thriving since 2010, but only because neighbors truck in water during the warm months. Some weeks, Hoselton has to drive to other garden sites to use their spigots. He fills fifty-gallon tubs and then hauls the water back up the hill in his Ford Explorer. Other gardeners fill buckets from their kitchen taps. "It'd sure be nice to have water here," one woman said. "It's not easy trucking three gallons of water and a baby."[6]

The water woes that plague Gilman Gardens are not unique. Water is perennially the number one concern with community gardeners. Running a water line to a garden site is a quick construction project that could return years of value to the community. Seattle's Department of Transportation could not stay on top of the maintenance of their street medians. And the lack of maintenance drives down property values. The Queen Anne neighborhood has absolved the City of this burden, saving the agency money and making Gilman Drive West a more desirable address.

The City argues providing water for gardens is complicated. It is not. Toilets, drinking fountains, display fountains, lawn sprinklers, and spray grounds are routinely supplied in public parks without cost to visitors. Supplying water to a garden is nothing for the municipality; but it is everything to the gardener.

If municipalities just cannot provide water to a site, there are alternatives to having gardeners truck in their own. One alternative is to steer urban agriculture to public land that is already irrigated.

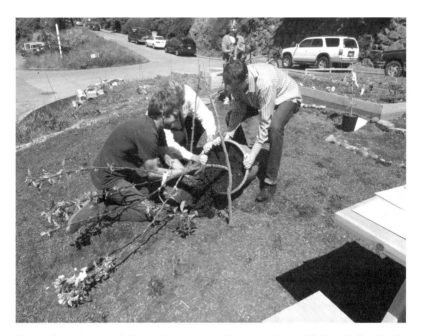

The author, along with King County Councilmember Larry Phillips, help Charlie Hoselton plant an apple tree on opening day of the Gilman Gardens.

In many parts of the country that do not receive adequate rainfall during the growing season (California, Texas, the Southwest, and some places in the Midwest, for example) the landscaping in public spaces might already be irrigated. Here, mixing edibles among the ornamentals ensures that the produce receives clean and ample watering. If the desired food-bearing plants are especially thirsty, plant them adjacent to lawns. Turf areas are heavily irrigated, and there is generally sufficient overspray to water the nearest plants.[7]

Selecting site-suitable plants also reduces maintenance and irrigation needs. Some plants are naturally labor intensive, while others thrive with little attention. One of the easiest ways to reduce maintenance demands is to select plants that are native or well suited to the particular geography of the city. Native plants often thrive without supplemental water, can effectively ward off indigenous pests (while attracting beneficial critters), and are generally less troublesome than crops foreign to an area. When plants are selected based on their natural suitability to a given locale, the natural order of things shoulders much of the maintenance, creating a productive and easier-to-care-for landscape.

There is also a great disparity in maintenance demands between woody perennials and herbaceous annuals. Teva Dawson, former community garden coordinator for the City of Des Moines and an active proponent of the municipality's goal to ensure food security in the city, found better success with food-producing woody perennials. Dawson learned that trees and shrubs only need care and supplemental water for the first couple of years to get established. After that, maintenance is minimal, thus providing a logical choice for municipalities with strained resources.[8] Most vegetables, with the exceptions of rhubarb, asparagus, and a handful of other, more exotic varieties, are annuals that require considerable care during the growing season, and will not live to see the next. By contrast, fruit and nuts are produced in abundance on a single tree, without the need for weeding, fertilizing, or supplemental water. Year after year, trees and shrubs produce without transplantation, replacement, or soil reconditioning. Some years may be less prolific than others; nevertheless, a single fruit or nut tree can supply food for many individuals.

Gail Savina agrees. In fact, Savina has a bit of a beef with the vegetable focus of urban agriculture. "Everyone talks about providing food for the community, yet so many are focused only on vegetables," Savina laments. "If we really are focused on substantive food—you know, *calories*—we would be planting more fruit trees." Savina's point is that fruit-bearing woody perennials are, calorie for calorie, and pound for pound, more cost-effective. In addition, "The footprint of a single fruit tree is nothing compared to the amount of space you would need to produce the same quantity of food with vegetables," she notes. Savina and I then talked about how folks typically measure success when growing food, and one yardstick is the total weight of the harvest. I mentioned to her that most gardening groups would be ecstatic if they could harvest, say, 1,000 pounds of vegetables over the course of a year. Savina quipped, "I can get that in a couple of days from a few fruit trees." Point well taken.

The difference in maintenance demands between vegetables and fruits aside, there is one concern that affects both equally: pests. Effectively managing pests in the landscape, even if chemical pesticides are used, can be a time-consuming endeavor for maintenance crews. So, why not let plants take on some of that burden? With a bit of plant knowledge, it is easier to manage troublesome bugs and critters without having to place additional demands on maintenance staff.

Mixing edibles with ornamentals is a great way to garden organically by naturally managing pests. Picking plants that attract beneficial critters while repelling malevolent ones is known as companion planting. It is one effective strategy within the environmentally sustainable process known as integrated pest management. In the city, where there is typically a strong desire for aesthetically pleasing and artfully composed landscapes, companion planting is a no-brainer.

One showy plant commonly used in the urban landscape is the marigold. Marigolds are quite effective at deterring all sorts of critters. Their vibrant blossoms are quite attractive to humans, but their unpleasant scent deters aphids, squirrels, thrips, squash bugs, and other pests. Marigolds also release a toxin in the soil that kills nematodes, but is safe for humans.

Artemesia, or wormwood, is quite effective in deterring many animals and foliage-devouring slugs. Some plants attract beneficial predator insects that, in turn, devour pesky ones. Alyssum and yarrow attract parasitoid wasps and hoverflies, which prey on spider mites, green flies, and small caterpillars. The plants need not be purely ornamental to deter pests. Plants with pungent scents and spicy flavors are quite effective at repelling unwanted critters, including rodents. Rosemary, onion, peppers, peppermint, garlic, thyme, chives, basil, cilantro, and other piquant herbs and vegetables keep scores of plant-devouring critters in check. Fennel repels fleas, sage repels slugs, and lavender repels mice and moths. It is a miraculous irony that the scents and flavors that are so compelling to people are so repulsive to pests; nature's insurance that we humans can eat, and eat well.

Mixing edibles with ornamentals not only is a marvelous way to reduce maintenance demands but also can ameliorate concerns over aesthetics. Many contend that vegetable gardens and fruit orchards provide an inappropriate look to our public places. We have become a culture where we expect our urban landscapes to be well groomed. Edible landscapes can be a bit unkempt and, because of that appearance, raise aesthetic objection by some. In the urban environment, it is arguably aesthetics alone that drive the plant palette in landscape design. Talented landscape architects and garden designers, however, weigh a litany of criteria when crafting a plant list. Some criteria are aesthetics, such as seasonal color, texture, and overall size of each plant for its particular site. But other criteria include environmental concerns, such as drought tolerance or erosion resistance; public safety and comfort (e.g., shrubs that block views from the street, trees that cast lots of shade, or plants with lots of prickly thorns); symbolism and cultural meaning; and, of course, maintenance. All of these concerns, and others, are balanced to enhance public spaces and add value for its users. Still, many lay people place aesthetics highest on the list of criteria considered, especially if the landscape is to accentuate a high-profile civic building.

Such a battle between beauty and bounty recently erupted in Baltimore. For years, the grounds outside of City Hall were planted with incredibly showy flowers. But in 2009, the landscape changed. Instead of daffodils and tulips, the Parks Department, working with the community's Master Gardeners, planted corn and tomatoes, beans and broccoli, beets, carrots, squash, peppers and eggplant, chard, kale, lettuce, and other leafy greens. The veggie garden was even designed by a landscape architect, to ensure the color, texture, and pattern of the garden maintained an appearance befitting the stature of City Hall.

The garden was a success by every measure. There were no vandals or varmints. The beds were lush and productive, yielding thousands of pounds of vegetables for the local soup kitchen. "I think it is really cool that the homeless are eating better than most of the citizens in the city of Baltimore," quipped the garden designer.[9] Passersby would stop and gawk at the produce, admitting they had never seen some of these vegetables outside the supermarket. It seemed everyone was happy.

Except for the mayor, who preferred the tulips.

During 2012, Baltimore's City Hall garden was drastically scaled back. In 2013, a few potato plants were all that remained from the once lengthy menu of vegetables. By 2014, even the potatoes were omitted. It was said that budget constraints were the sole factor in the demise of the vegetable garden. Though the Master Gardeners will tell you they are volunteers, and cared for the vegetable garden *pro bono*. Not only that, but the seeds for all the vegetables were donated by a local seed company.

But at the end of the day, one wonders if some important public officials didn't think vegetables were important enough for this public site. Chief of Horticulture Melissa Grim admitted, "Making vegetables look pretty in such a formal, high-profile site is tricky."[10]

High-ranking officials in the capital of Vermont, however, do see tremendous beauty in vegetables. In fact, they consider vegetables so stately that they deserve a place in the State House front lawn.

Montpelier, like other municipalities throughout the country, felt the economic pinch of 2009. The Great Recession forced deep budget cuts across all Montpelier's programs, including cuts to the State House front yard. There simply was no money left to maintain a showy landscape; flowers were deemed fiscally imprudent. The State budget—as reflected in the grounds—was bleak.

But certainly a historic property with such civic significance deserves the attention and grandeur of a nice landscape. Local citizens agreed. So a few dedicated individuals got together and formed the APPLE Corps, the Association for the Planting of Public edible Landscapes for Everyone. Their mission? To return splendor to the State House front lawn, while espousing their belief that "the presence of vegetables, herbs, and fruit and nut trees in public spaces can help educate people about local food, while enhancing our food security."[11]

State officials in coats and ties, kneeling on the ground with more casually dressed APPLE Corps members planted chard, beets, red cabbage, sage, and lettuces—plants high in both nutritional and aesthetic value. "Our intention is to create a garden there that is not only edible and educational, but that fits in with the beauty, aesthetics, balance and symmetry already found on the State House lawn," noted one APPLE Corps-er.[12]

The group succeeded admirably. Not only was the new edible landscape a thing of beauty, but it produced 600 pounds of vegetables in the first two years (most of that bulk from leafy greens!). The soup kitchen chefs, tourists to the State House, government officials, and the community at-large were all quite pleased with the new face of the front lawn.

There is no doubt that food-producing plants can be messy and need some upkeep. But the pervasive assumption that edibles require considerably *more* management than ornamental plants, or are not as pretty, is bogus. Sure, intensive row-crop agriculture in our public parks is probably a maintenance headache, and may not be desirable within some urban settings. A challenge that befits the astute public-space designer is incorporating edibles into a successful park or plaza design. Just as one would not plant large, thorny shrubs like firethorn and cactus next to a playground for toddlers, so too should a measure of caution be exercised when planting edibles. In other words, sound design principles are not

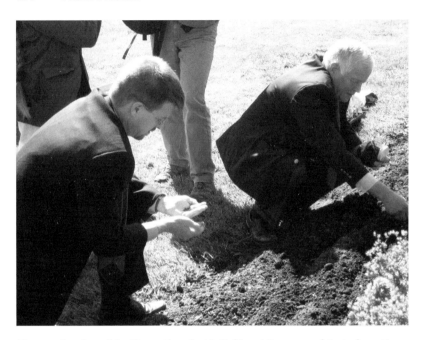

Vermont Speaker of the House Shap Smith (left) and Secretary of Agriculture Roger Allbee plant vegetable seeds on the State House front lawn. (Courtesy of Glenn Scherer)

thrown out the window simply because the plant palette uses fruit-bearing trees instead of sterile cultivars. As in any landscape design, the architect needs to take into account how many people will use or pass by the space; what types of activities will take place in the space; the microclimate, solar access, and water availability of the space; and a host of other variables. When planting our backyard garden, we often do not consider these variables. We know we want pole beans, potatoes, radishes, maybe some carrots, and "Oh! We *have* to have tomatoes!" (What garden is complete without tomatoes?), maybe some lettuces, and, what the heck, let's try some watermelon. There is little thought given to the garden's aesthetic composition, and there is no need to consider who else might be using the space, since it is in our backyard. This type of edible landscape is inappropriate in many public settings. A better,

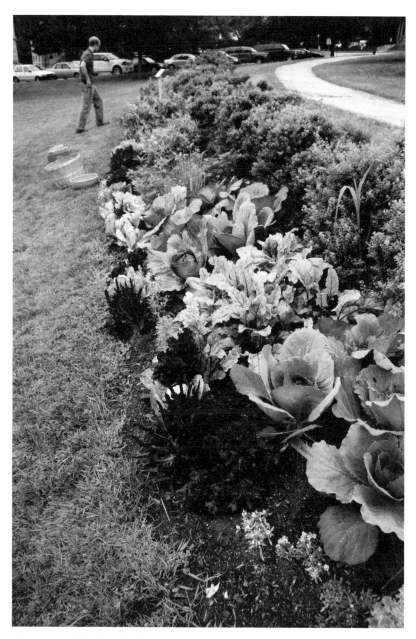

Blue-green collards, red cabbage, beet greens, and rainbow chard provide colorful —and edible—adornment to the State House landscape in Montpelier. (Courtesy of Annie Tiberio Cameron)

more balanced approach is to mix edibles with ornamentals, something we don't typically see in backyard gardens. This means roses with tomatoes, rosemary and citrus mixed with fortnight lily, fennel mixed with purple fountain grass, persimmon and cherry trees interspersed with dogwoods, for example—all within a park or plaza setting that attracts users with beauty and offers opportunities for social and physical sustenance.

A fantastic example of an edible landscape imbued with artistry and beauty was recently created in New York City. Once a beleaguered community garden up for auction, the space was spared and miraculously transformed with the help of two music sensations who, on the surface, couldn't be more dissimilar.

Rap-sensation Curtis "50-Cent" Jackson and mega-entertainer Bette Midler teamed up together in Jamaica, Queens, over their love of fresh produce. That and to create a public gathering spot brimming with social activity and neighborhood pride. For Jackson, underwriting the garden renovation was a way to give back to his boyhood home. Midler is the founder of the New York Restoration Project (NYRP), a group that works to clean and restore various park spaces and community gardens in the city. And this particular garden—dilapidated and located in a neighborhood in sore need of quality open space—was well deserving of the attention from two international celebrities.

Midler's group kick-started the transformation by asking the gardeners what improvements they would like to see. The executive director of NYRP recalled that "none of them liked the way the gardens looked. In some cases, all they wanted was something simple, like a more attractive fence, but in others, they wanted a new design that would make the space feel more open and welcoming." Walter Hood, a gifted landscape architect recognized for his design of bold, sculptural urban spaces, was then chosen for the renovation. What Hood created was something few community gardeners had ever seen.

Linden trees with an understory of carpet roses announce the garden's entrance, while an arbor covered with trumpet vines runs along the garden's length. Inside the garden, raised vegetable beds are laid in parallel lines, a nod to the rail line that runs alongside the northeast edge of the site. French-styled parterres create formal spaces where boxwood surrounds heirloom vegetables, pumpkins, corn, and other edibles. And perhaps the most striking elements of the garden are the half dozen, ten-foot-tall rainwater collectors that resemble giant blue martini glasses. These colorful collectors funnel 3,000 gallons of rainwater to two underground cisterns, providing not only a convenient and ecologically friendly water source for the gardeners, but a celebratory element that attracts attention from all passersby. Hood notes, "I was trying to find something that might capture the imagination." It seems he has succeeded. One resident exclaimed, "To me, it's the most beautiful site. All I want is to just sit and absorb it."[13]

For those *still* skeptical about the suitability of fruits and vegetables in ornamental landscapes, perhaps a trip to Tomorrowland will convince you. Recent visitors to Disneyland do double takes at the carpets of herbs and leafy greens surrounding the Astro Orbiter. Walk a few more paces and you find still more fruits and vegetables in the shadow of the elevated monorail. Citrus, chard, bok choy, thyme, variegated sage, and red leaf lettuce are planted in bold masses and striking patterns, creating interesting contrasts in texture and color. The design is well crafted, as you would expect from Disney's imagineers. Though the first glance at these grounds takes park visitors (including me) by surprise, after a second look, the gardens seem wholly appropriate for the Happiest Place on Earth.

These edible landscapes are not just another whimsical display from the designers at Disneyland. There is a prescient message hidden in these garden beds. It is no coincidence Disney's landscapers chose Tomorrowland to plant food in lieu of flowers. Striking landscapes, embellished with vivid splashes of orange, lemon yellow, and cherry red—titillating our eyes as well as our tongues—are the landscapes of the future.

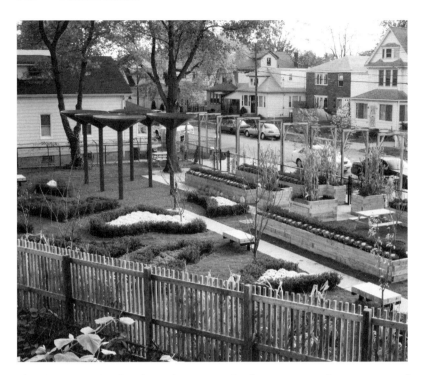

The Curtis "50 Cent" Jackson Community Garden is a stunning composition of forms, colors, and textures accomplished with the help of vegetables. (Courtesy of the New York Restoration Project)

To the chagrin of architects, planners, and landscape and urban designers, maintenance often drives the design of our buildings and the spaces between them. Rather than this skewed approach, the designs of our human settlements first need to consider the needs of their inhabitants, and then bring into play programs and strategies to help ensure those needs are met and maintained. As has become obvious, I am offering successful strategies to help quell the fears of municipal officials who have long discouraged— or outright forbidden—the use of edibles in our urban landscapes, solely because of maintenance and aesthetic concerns.

I do not mean to diminish the importance of maintenance and aesthetics in our public places. Beauty inspires us, and proper

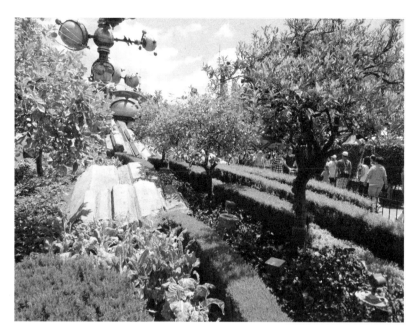

Orange trees, clipped herbs, and salad greens greet visitors to Tomorrowland, symbolizing the ornamental landscapes of the future.

maintenance plays a significant role in the attractiveness of space. But these considerations should be balanced with the greater good that providing the community with food choices offers. What typically adorn our urban landscapes are trees and shrubs that are high in aesthetic value, low in food value, and yet similar with regard to maintenance requirements as comparable edibles. What should be weighed is the added value certain plants provide to users of public space vis-à-vis the perceived added burdens of maintenance. When properly selected, edibles as landscape plants have the ability to achieve all the public-safety, comfort, aesthetics, drought-tolerance, and general maintenance goals required of plants in public space, with one notable addition: they help establish food security.

Chapter 6

Food Literacy

Peanuts do not grow on trees, nor do pineapples. Green bell peppers are underripe red bell peppers. Parsnips are not related to parsley, but they are related to carrots. Not all potatoes come from Idaho. Ask a nine-year-old where an apple comes from, and he or she will likely respond, "The grocery store."

Americans today are food illiterate. For a nation rooted in agrarianism, it is frightening how ignorant of food we have become. Our Big Ag brand of food production has given us unprecedented convenience, from fast-food and prepackaged meals (so that we do not have to learn to cook) to year-round mangoes and asparagus (so that we do not have to worry about what grows in our corner of the world or at what time).

Public produce can help us regain that great agrarian knowledge our forefathers possessed. The trees, shrubs, rambling vines, and showy annuals we choose to adorn our streets, parks, plazas, and city squares can offer visual delight as well as lessons on healthy eating. But we need to get back to basics. A growing number of Americans have never seen fruits and vegetables in their native habitat, much less plucked them from the vine.

Once we start seeding our public landscapes with fresh produce, we will have to learn how to distinguish food from ornamentals (and remember they can be both). We will have to learn what parts of a plant are edible, and which are not (rhubarb, for example, has toxic leaves; only the petioles, the red stalks, should be eaten). We will have to learn when to expect those fruits and vegetables (apples in autumn, citrus in winter, asparagus in spring, and summer squash in, well, you get the idea). And we will have to learn to appreciate those forgotten foods that were once commonly enjoyed, but have disappeared from our diet (like juneberries, hickory nuts, and pawpaw) as well as the culturally diverse foods that more accurately reflect the eating habits of our melting pot nation.

Bolstering the depth and breadth of our food knowledge is a daunting endeavor. But getting back to basics doesn't mean municipal employees have to create a food curriculum from scratch, or become experts themselves. Municipal budgets are lean, and I know from experience just how tight city staff are stretched. Luckily, public officials can draw from the knowledge and passion of others in their community to help citizens become more food literate. Gardening clubs, zealous parents and teachers, farmers' markets, and nonprofit groups committed to locally grown produce and healthy eating reside in every community, and each can partner with the municipality to help lessen our food ignorance.

One of the best examples of this partnering strategy can be found in Kamloops, British Columbia. The Kamloops Food Policy Council (KFPC) is a nonprofit advocacy group that works with municipal leaders to educate the public on community food security. Through public presentations, gardening workshops, and even cooking demonstrations, KFPC is able to teach citizens about food and healthy eating, while weaving in strategies to address larger food policy issues. The organization also helps establish concrete food system projects, like community gardens and an urban gleaning program, similar to City Fruit in Seattle. But the most innovative of KFPC's projects is the Public Produce Program, which just might be a veggie lover's Xanadu.

When the Program started in 2011, the first public produce garden was located smack in the middle of downtown, amid the hubbub and bustle of Victoria Street. Colorful wooden planter boxes, benches, and an artfully crafted trellis created what looked to be an alfresco produce market, but where the tomatoes, eggplant, and mizuna lettuce grew in situ. Also unlike the typical produce market, these vegetables were free, the only cost being your willingness to harvest the food yourself.

The crops were kept tidy by Master Gardeners and other community volunteers, who also encouraged passersby to help themselves. Folks usually had questions about the garden in general as well as a particular vegetable that was unfamiliar to them. The volunteers taught them about the different varieties while explaining how public produce can bolster food security. Of course, the volunteers couldn't be there round the clock to pass on their knowledge to passersby, so they drafted artful signs informing folks when radishes were ready to harvest or the proper manner of picking bush beans, for example. Fun and educational celebrations were held from time to time in the garden, and suddenly, downtown had a new convivial gathering space—one that nourished body, mind, and soul.

"This pilot project was extraordinarily successful," notes KFPC's website, in large measure because it was so readily embraced by the community.[1] People are obviously drawn to fresh produce, and KFPC's location for the public produce garden could not have been more suitable. The vegetables and the benches beckon the hundreds who amble by daily to sit a spell and learn a bit about food and healthy eating.

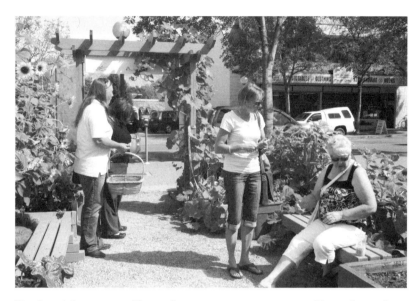

Kamloops' downtown public produce project is one part vegetable garden and one part community gathering space, which yields a fantastic learning environment. (Courtesy of Kendra Besanger)

But the extraordinary success of this public produce garden is not because downtown Kamloopsians enjoy fresh produce more than their compatriots. Public produce is successful in Kamloops because it is in the public consciousness, thanks to KFPC's tireless advocacy. The group printed posters and passed them out around town, announcing the arrival of the public produce gardens. Presentations were given to various community groups and municipal staff. Television and newspaper reporters were invited to cover the public produce efforts. KFPC created a blog and a Facebook page to announce various public produce events, post sumptuous pictures of ripe produce, and offer lessons on growing food and healthy eating. They even published what I would call the definitive *How To* guide for public produce. This inspiring manual—written by Elaine Sedgman, a Master Gardener and cocreator of Kamloops' public produce gardens—offers lessons and expert insights any municipality on any continent would find useful.

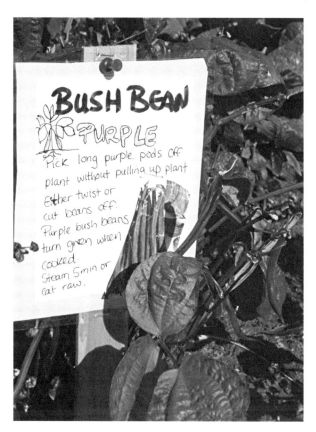

Fun signs like this teach us not only about different vegetables but about how to harvest and eat them. (Courtesy of Erin Edwards and Elaine Sedgman)

Because the value of public produce became so apparent to the community, the gardens have spread. Public vegetables have been planted in front of City Hall; in decorative sidewalk planters along Victoria Street; on a vacant parcel in a residential neighborhood; and in two city parks. KFPC taught the community and civic leaders about the value of public fruits and vegetables, and the organization used every conduit for information at their disposal to deliver their message.

Many of those conduits, however, were provided by the municipality. As part of an ongoing community education plan, KFPC notes they will rely on "the expertise of the City of Kamloops' horticultural, media and marketing, environmental and irrigation staff." Educational seminars are published on the city's website and in community activity guides. KFPC is also thankful the municipality will help "with environmental education and assist where necessary through their environmental services and sustainability departments."[2]

The Kamloops Public Produce Program demonstrates the ingenuity required to educate a community about better food choices. The content of a food literacy curriculum—knowing what food is and where it comes from, who is growing it and how, when it is ready to harvest, and why this knowledge matters—is crucial to alleviating food insecurity. But content alone isn't particularly useful; consumers need to be able to find it easily, read it, and get excited about it. So how can municipalities large and small organize food literacy programs that effectively reach their citizens?

Strategies for creating *and* disseminating information to the masses may be quite similar to those employed during the victory garden campaign of World War II. For that effort, the government exploited every media outlet available at the time. Promotional and educational articles were published in local newspapers and popular gardening magazines; audio clips and short films were created and broadcast to the community via radio and classroom projectors; and mimeograph technology allowed pamphlets, handouts, and bulletins to be widely distributed. The abundant and comprehensive information ranged from planting techniques to suggestions on which vegetables provided the greatest nutrition, variety, and utility. Recipes, information on canning and preserving, and other preparation and storage tips were also provided, along with methods to extend the growing season and maximize yields. Indeed, the entire structure of the victory garden program was formed around the efficient dissemination of information.[3]

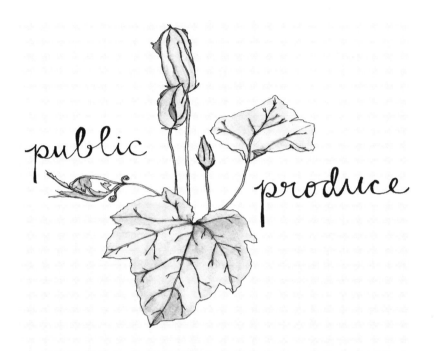

GROWING FOOD IN PUBLIC SPACES

A START UP GUIDE

KAMLOOPS FOOD POLICY COUNCIL

This Kamloops How To *guide provides invaluable lessons to any municipality interested in establishing a public produce program. The guide is available through the Kamloops Food Policy Council website: http://kamloopsfoodpolicycouncil.com/. (Courtesy of Elaine Sedgman)*

Today, the challenge is much the same, but the conduits for information are far superior. Government-access television allows municipalities to create custom television programs tailored for their community. A creative communications department could tap the skills of the municipality's horticulture staff, and produce fun and informative television segments on pruning fruit trees, or distinguishing chard from kale. Printed material, such as Fallen Fruit's neighborhood fruit tree maps, can be included with monthly utility bills or city newsletters. And gardening courses—already commonly offered through parks and recreation departments—could be expanded to include cooking demonstrations utilizing public produce.

As Kamloops discovered, the greatest advancement in disseminating information lies in the virtual world. Social media sites like Facebook and Twitter allow municipalities and community groups to send food tips and tidbits to thousands of people directly and instantly, with little cost or effort expended. The City's website or blog can host instructional videos and informational downloads that can be accessed anytime. The City doesn't even have to create the content themselves. Restaurateurs, gardening groups, and food bloggers are usually more than happy to lend recipes and ideas from their own websites to others who find them useful. It's a win-win, as the municipality doesn't have to spend time writing new content, and the others get broad recognition for their efforts. Indeed, a well-designed, content-rich website could provide unparalleled virtual instruction in a compelling and fun manner.

The nonprofit Center for Urban Education about Sustainable Agriculture (CUESA) has a website full of great ideas that municipalities could easily adapt for their own purposes. CUESA, which manages San Francisco's Ferry Plaza farmers' market, packs its website chock-a-block with all sorts of food and agricultural content in a mouthwatering manner. From the Glossary page, which succinctly teaches the difference between *heirloom*, *heritage*, and *hybrid*, to the A to Z Sustainability Guide, CUESA offers provocative content paired with delicious photography, infused with soul-enriching philosophy.

For me, CUESA's most valuable online resource is their seasonality charts, which I think of as fruit, nut, and vegetable calendars. These charts help consumers better understand their agricultural geography, by teaching them what grows where when. Bay Area consumers can find out just when those prized California artichokes, pistachios, or fava beans are available at the Ferry Plaza farmers' market by logging on to cuesa.org. These calendars also list a variety of unusual crops that reflect both the ethnic diversity and the adventurous foodie spirit that prevail in San Francisco. Produce such as cactus pads and pears, cardoons, burdock, salsify, feijoas, jujubes, and cherimoyas are listed among the more familiar avocados, fennel, figs, bok choy, shallots, and tomatillos.

Of course, California's mild climate enables a tantalizing array of food to be grown throughout the year. But it is just as important for South Dakotans to understand what grows in their neck of the woods and when it is ripe, so that they, too, can cultivate an interest in food and appreciation for the unique environment in which they live.

What makes CUESA's website so appealing even to the supermarket shopper is marketing: the design of the site, the enticing descriptions of ripe fruit, and the photographs of smiling, happy people. Make no mistake, CUESA is a business like any other. Marketing is about getting consumers excited about your product, and for CUESA, their product is locally grown produce. For public produce to succeed, citizens across the community have to feel the same excitement for locally grown fruits and vegetables that Bay Area residents feel when they visit CUESA's website. Improving literacy is far easier when students are giddy over the subject matter.

I recall one brilliant example of marketing in the produce aisle of a popular supermarket in Chapel Hill, North Carolina. It was winter, and the store was filled with fresh citrus (unfortunately, from all over the world, but that's not my point). Most Americans know just four types of citrus: oranges, lemons, limes, and grapefruit. But what about pomelos and kumquats?

The supermarket, recognizing that consumers won't buy things they are unfamiliar with, created a huge, eye-catching display. The colorful chart was hung above the citrus stand, in a location you really had to make an effort to ignore. It was a simple yet compelling display, coercing consumers into learning about the different types of citrus.

Within a few moments, shoppers could easily identify a kumquat, a pomelo, and a tangelo. The chart also explained how to select and store each particular citrus fruit. This sort of education has immense value to consumers, as it encourages diversity in their diets. But it also has value to the supermarket, as it encouraged us consumers to buy produce we otherwise wouldn't have given a second look to. (I bought my first pomelo that day.) This is a valuable marketing tactic and educational lesson for anyone desiring to promote public produce. Fear is the brood of ignorance, and we are generally apprehensive of the unfamiliar—whether it is an unknown fruit or the idea of harvesting dinner ingredients from the side of the street. A little education goes a long way to encourage acceptance of the once unknown, and such educational material can pique our curiosity and help develop an appreciation for diverse fruits and vegetables.

Part of a successful system of public produce is providing diverse foods to our diverse citizens. Learning about new fruits and vegetables is like learning new words in our language. In our multicultural North American cities, expanding our food vocabulary is also good for community and culture. Vegetables and fruits you may not like (or even recognize as food) might be highly prized by your neighbors. In order to provide public space edibles for all members of the public, we have to step back and consider, "Just what is food?"

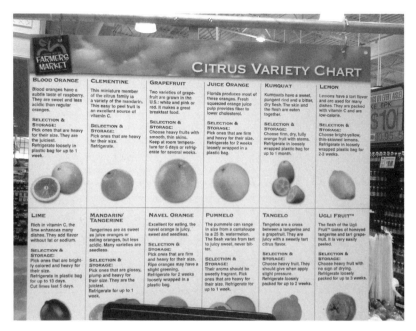

This attractive and informative display helps shoppers in Chapel Hill, North Carolina, recognize, select, and store assorted varieties of citrus.

Take dandelions, for example. These weeds are the scourge of suburban homeowners everywhere. But dandelion greens are a delicious and nutritious addition to any garden salad, and shockingly command a pretty hefty price at the farmers' market. Purslane, sometimes referred to as pigweed, is as denigrated as the dandelion. Yet this succulent provides a pleasing crunch to any salad, and it is also packed with nutrients. (Want omega-3s in your diet but you don't eat fish? Try purslane. It has more omega-3 fatty acids than any other leafy vegetable!) Chickweed is another fantastic food that folks want to annihilate rather than celebrate. Chayote climbs with reckless abandon in the mild-winter states of the country, but yields wholesome gourds revered by many. Nasturtiums spread like wildfire, but both the leaves and flowers provide pretty—and peppery—accompaniments to any meal. Many plants

have tremendous value as food crops, but because we have perceived them for so long as weeds, we may not recognize them as
food at all.

To help folks gain an appreciation of the myriad edible plants
in their environment that can be found wild, or those that can be
cultivated for food, public officials may want to include recipes
with other food information they publish or circulate. The suburban homeowner that has cursed dandelions for years might have a
difficult time believing that those vexing plants are actually prized
salad greens. But one taste and skeptics could become believers.

CUESA's website hosts an extensive recipe database that could
give inspiration to municipalities and food advocacy groups interested in enticing folks to try different foods. Visitors to the site can
search for recipes based on season (spring, summer, fall, or winter) or type of preparation (entrée, dessert, appetizers, drinks). The
website will then return a menu of delectable dishes that highlight
seasonal produce, some with ingredients we typically regard as
weeds. For example, search for *spring* and *soup* and CUESA returns
recipes like purslane, chilled cucumber, and buttermilk soup;
stinging nettle soup; and spring sorrel soup. Sound scrumptious?
Keep in mind these aren't foul-tasting concoctions from some well-
intentioned but culinary-challenged naturalist. These recipes are
from professional chefs in the Bay Area; dishes so tasty people pay
good money for them. Yet they utilize plants most wouldn't even
think were food.

An extensive food vocabulary is crucial to ensure food security—
both in being able to produce a bounty of food regardless of one's
landscape and to preserve cultures and traditions of our many ethnic families. Food security is commonly defined as "access to nutritious, affordable, safe, adequate, and *culturally acceptable* food on a
daily basis."[4] For homogenous countries, like Finland and Japan,
culturally acceptable is more tightly defined and commonly under-
stood. But in our multicultural melting pot, culturally acceptable

food means a greater variety than is offered through the more typical fresh-produce outlets. As Mark Winne notes, "Many CSAs and farmers who sell at farmers' markets are responding only to the food preferences of an educated, white clientele. To be inclusive of a more racially and ethnically diverse customer base, farmers—most of whom are white—have to learn how to grow crops preferred by nonwhite customers."[5]

The need for culturally acceptable produce is perhaps one of the greatest reasons why a central government policy on food will ultimately fail the food security test. Centralized policies, regardless of their reform aims, tend to be of a one-size-fits-all mold. Such a policy regarding food would likely erase the unique traditions and customs of our celebrated ethnic diversity expressed through food and cuisine, replacing them with a more homogenous menu of food items. Food literacy has much to do with an understanding of culture and ethnic diversity, and which foods have meaning and value to the diverse racial groups that comprise our communities. The common globe eggplant, for example, is not suitable for the Chinese, who prefer their own, more slender, delicately flavored variety. Likewise, people of Japanese, Indian, Italian, and other cultures prize specific varieties of eggplant, some of which are not readily available in US supermarkets. Thai eggplants, with their green striped color and spherical shape, bear little resemblance to the common globe eggplant, and are perhaps the most difficult to source. But they are essential to authentic Thai cuisine.

In most instances, culturally acceptable food is not simply a different variety of more common produce items, but foods that white Americans simply would not recognize as food at all. Ginkgo nuts, for instance, are revered by Chinese, Korean, and Japanese families. However, in the United States, the prevailing (i.e., non-Asian) sentiment is that the fruit-producing female trees should be avoided at all costs, as the aromas of crushed ginkgo fruits remind many of an unsavory amalgamation of canine feces, rancid butter, and vomit.

Certainly not pleasant—and, for this reason, many people have ardently sought to remove female ginkgo trees from city spaces. But the ginkgo nuts are quite tasty, and almost impossible to find in any market outside of Chinatown. The solution, a rather simple but effective one, is to harvest the ginkgo fruit before they fall to the ground and are crushed by unappreciative feet. For folks living on the East Coast, where ginkgoes are found in great abundance, it is common to see people of Asian descent—often elderly Chinese women—gathering the ginkgo fruit.

Prickly pear cactus is a spiny, robust plant with high ornamental value to white Americans for their water-conserving gardens. But to Mexican families, *nopales* is a staple in their traditional cuisine. Callaloo (amaranth greens) is a much sought-after leafy green vegetable in African-Caribbean communities, though few other cultures have developed a taste for it.

Of course, context is vital to the success of public produce. Female ginkgo trees may be unwelcome in predominantly white suburbs of America. Callaloo would likely be regarded as a weed. Prickly pear may be more acceptable, but only as a specimen in a xeriscape garden. But when certain fruits that are deemed unpalatable to others are planted where citizens not only recognize them as food, but prize them because they are part of their rich cultural heritage—and because they cannot be found through the typical food outlets—they add immense value to public space, and to the city as a whole.

We also need to recognize that ethnic food that was at one time foreign has now become (or is capable of becoming) culturally acceptable to the masses, including white America. Not too long ago in California, for example, bok choy and daikon radish were virtually unheard of except in Asian markets, and could have been deemed, at the time, culturally unacceptable to many Americans. During the late 1980s, however, the popularity of Asian vegetables skyrocketed—almost overnight. Between 1988 and 1989, the production of Asian vegetables in California increased 41 percent.[6]

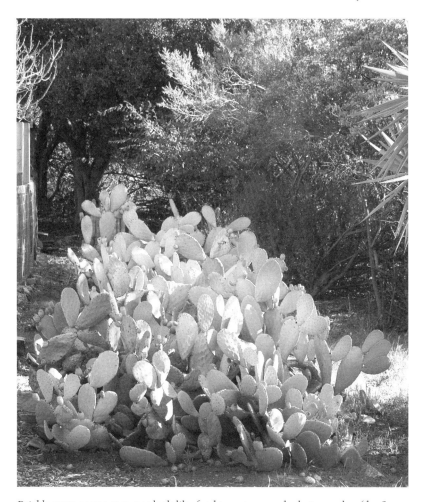

Prickly pear cactus may not look like food to many people, but nopales *(the Spanish name for the large, flat pads) and* tuna *(the prickly pear fruits atop the pads) are highly regarded in Mexican communities and are a staple in authentic Mexican and New Mexican cuisine.*

Today, bok choy and daikon radish are readily found in supermarkets throughout the state (indeed, throughout the country!), enjoyed by Chinese, Hispanics, blacks, and whites. Chinese cuisine has become immensely popular in America, as has Japanese, Indian, Mexican, Ethiopian, Thai, Vietnamese, Caribbean, and

Greek, illustrating that foods that are still typically regarded as culturally "foreign" can also be highly desirable.

In the United States, where diversity is celebrated, culturally acceptable foods open a world of gustatory opportunity, while addressing issues of food security. For this very reason, municipal staff in Des Moines purposely planted produce varieties that are quite unfamiliar to Iowans. Some examples found throughout the city's many edible landscapes include jostaberry, pawpaw, medlar, Asian pear, Chinese chestnut, and juneberry. As Teva Dawson of the city's Parks and Recreation Department noted, "It was very important for us to choose some varieties that we knew were hardy and disease resistant as well as more unique and unusual plant varieties that folks would not find in their grocery store."[7] Obviously we need to ensure apples, pears, plums, attractive leafy greens and other recognizable staples are provided within our edible landscapes. But we also need to become more food fluent, and what is necessary are programs that teach the public how to harvest, prepare, and eat foods such as loquat, carob, sorrel, nasturtium, fennel, dandelion, chayote, prickly pear, jujube, passion fruit, feijoa, and a host of other vegetables and fruits that our ethnic communities (and a growing number of restaurateurs, for that matter) across the nation prize.

As we accept a more varied menu of food choices, landscape architects, as the principal designers of urban open space, will have to sharpen their agricultural acumen as well. Seasoned landscape architects have committed to memory hundreds of trees, shrubs, and groundcovers—their botanical names as well as their common ones. The vast majority of their plant knowledge, however, is lopsidedly focused on ornamentals. Currently, edible landscapes are a niche market for the few landscape designers who wish to take it on. In the future, it will no longer be a niche. Landscape architects will need to be versed in ornamental and edible plants, and how to plant them in combinations that create not only beautiful compositions but compositions that realize the principles of integrated pest management and companion planting, while providing utility, joy, comfort, and relief to people in public space.

In Seattle, one team of landscape designers is already showcasing that future trend in their profession. In the culturally diverse neighborhood of Beacon Hill, an incredibly ambitious edible park is underway. I say ambitious because their public produce garden—if fully realized—will be the largest in the country on municipal land, and the lessons this garden will teach go far beyond fruit and vegetable basics.

The Beacon Food Forest is an inspiring transformation of underutilized public land. What was once seven acres of lonesome lawn entrapped behind a security fence to keep the public out is now a burgeoning outdoor classroom espousing the benefits of permaculture.

This innovative educational garden began as a classroom assignment in 2009. Glenn Herlihy and Jacqueline Cramer were two students in a permaculture design course, and the final project was a "dream design" that incorporated all the principles of permaculture. The pair chose a site surrounding Seattle's first public drinking water reservoir, a patch of land that sat idle for the better part of a century, fenced off from the Beacon Hill residents. As part of the assignment, Herlihy and Cramer presented their design to the neighborhood and the City of Seattle. Unlike most student projects that get shelved once the course is completed, their project caught the eye of the community.

Over the next couple of years, word had spread about this incredible landscape proposal, and community presentations became more frequent. The plans for the Beacon Food Forest called for a couple of acres of community gardens, another couple of acres of "open forage zone" (fruit and nut trees and shrubs, herbs, and vegetables free for anyone to harvest), and the last portion devoted to group teaching gardens. The City was skeptical but the public loved it.

In 2012, the security fence was removed and the land was turned over to the city's Parks and Recreation Department to manage a new community green space: Jefferson Park. Initially, plans for an arboretum were bandied about on the site of the food forest, but the community preferred Herlihy's and Cramer's permaculture concept. Finally, after more than three years of planning and community discussions, the first phase of the Beacon Food Forest was completed—two acres of the seven-acre site now house garden plots, blueberry shrubs, herbs, dozens of fruit trees, and, of course, space to teach the principles of permaculture.

By now you're probably asking, "What the heck is permaculture?" It is an ecological design philosophy pioneered by two Australian blokes in the 1970s. A Seattle-based journalist covering the Beacon Food Forest explains permaculture as . . .

> . . . an ecological design system, philosophy, and set of ethics and principles used to create perennial, self-sustaining landscapes and settlements that build ecological knowledge and skills in communities. The concept of a food forest is a core concept of permaculture design derived from wild food ecosystems, where land often becomes forest if left to its own devices. In a food forest, everything from the tree canopy to the roots is edible or useful in some way.[8]

At first blush, improving food access for the Beacon Hill residents seems to be the driving force behind the Beacon Food Forest. A park brimming with free public fruits and herbs is certainly enticing, and the community relishes the food-growing potential of their new neighborhood green space. But Herlihy's and Cramer's goals for the food forest are broader. When I asked Herlihy what he sees as the core mission behind a permaculture garden, he immediately replied, "Addressing nature deprivation, across the board."

Herlihy explained that he feels it is supremely important that the Beacon Food Forest teach urbanites about nature and habitat rehabilitation. And part of the lesson plan of habitat restoration is food education: "Where does food come from, and how does it get to my plate?" Increasing access to healthy food is an important tenet of the Beacon Food Forest. But it is just one tenet of four. "The Beacon Food Forest's mission can be summarized in four parts," Herlihy told me. "Build community. Educate community. Build a garden. Share food."[9]

The Beacon Food Forest's cocreator has a different take, however. While Herlihy is focused on nature, Cramer's focus *is* food security. Cramer has a farming background, and for her the driving motivator was cultivating underutilized public land to serve folks who can barely afford fresh fruits and vegetables.

Cramer sees the open forage zone as a way to not only improve food access to this working-class neighborhood, but also reinforce cultural traditions. She explained to me that there was concern that many ethnic families in Beacon Hill would see the project as "white folks making food for us."[10] Cramer worked to dispel that notion. She recognized that many families with Asian ancestry, for example, have no connection to their homeland through the produce that is typically available to them in the markets. So Cramer felt a diverse plant palette was critical. The Beacon Food Forest plans call for a host of Asian-native fruits, such as quince, persimmon, and Asian pear, chosen because they will grow quite well in the local climate, yet strengthen cultural ties to far away places.

Regardless of whether the focus is habitat rehabilitation or food security, the Beacon Food Forest offers great lessons in creating healthy and happy communities. Margarett Harrison, the lead landscape architect for the project, was quoted as saying, "If this is successful, it is going to set such a precedent for the city of Seattle, and for the whole Northwest."[11]

Harrison may have been modest in her estimation. If the Beacon Food Forest is successful—and early signs suggest it will be—it just might set a precedent for urban food production in the entire developed world.

As the Beacon Food Forest illustrates, the target audience of food literacy efforts is critical to the success of public produce. The educational gardens and strategies I just profiled, however, are all aimed at adult consumers: those who can choose what to eat and from where. But food education isn't just for grownups. In fact, the quickest way to become a food-literate nation once again is to teach our children the ways of the carrot and the strawberry.

Food literacy, like language, is most effective when it is taught at a young age, and many experts say food and dietary choices taught early in life set lifelong patterns. For these reasons, many communities have incorporated schoolyard gardens as part of the education curriculum.

Schoolyard gardens as public education have a long history in this country, dating back to the 1890s with the Putnam School in Boston. At that time there was great enthusiasm for public school gardens, and integrating gardening into the curricula was a national movement. According to community garden authority Laura Lawson, prominent figures of the time, like journalist Jacob Riis, landscape architect Frederick Law Olmsted, and a young political upstart named Woodrow Wilson, "praised gardening for its contributions to youngsters' education, health, industrial training, and general civic-mindedness." [12] In her book, *City Bountiful*, Lawson noted this:

> Concerns during this period about urban and rural conditions, child development, and civic improvement found a shared solution in school gardens. Because gardening was considered a means to address a range of educational, social, moral, recreational, and environmental agendas, children's garden programs enjoyed a broad base of support from teachers, government agencies, institutions, garden clubs, social reformers, and civic groups.[13]

But over the next 100 years, the popularity of public school gardening waxed and waned with the changing agricultural attitudes and economic times. Today, thankfully, schoolyard gardens are enjoying a renewed vigor, which could not be more timely, given the rise in childhood obesity and the preponderance in our children's diets of processed and fast foods—many of which, ironically, are available to kids in their school cafeterias.

As Lawson revealed, schoolyard gardens teach children basic life lessons, such as self-sufficiency, the natural cycles of life, and more rudimentary, where food comes from. Many children today have no idea that potatoes come from the ground, nuts from the tree, or grapes from the vine. Teaching kids to garden gives them a sense of accomplishment, while exposing them to a diversity of whole foods and the miracle of Mother Nature. Getting our kids interested in fresh fruits and vegetables will be the quickest manner to change our fast-food culture to a slow-food one. Most importantly, teaching children to garden establishes a pattern of healthy eating. As Ron Finley, the guerilla gardener from South Central discovered, "When children grow kale, children eat kale."[14]

Michael Pollan agrees. Pollan contends that we may never fully develop an appreciation and fondness for healthy foods until there is a significant change in our food culture. And that change, he says, "must begin with our children, and it must begin in our schools." Pollan maintains that eating well is a critical life skill, and that "we need to teach all primary-school students the basics of growing and cooking food." Much like President Kennedy recognized the woeful physical ability of our nation's children a half century ago—and then mandated physical education be established in public schools—many today, like Pollan, are arguing for an equally important "edible education."[15]

The most famous and comprehensive edible education program in the nation is found in Berkeley, at Martin Luther King Jr. Middle School. The Edible Schoolyard, the brainchild of Chez Panisse founder and slow-food advocate Alice Waters, is a one-acre organic garden and kitchen classroom. Before the garden was created, the grounds around the school comprised asphalt, parched turf, and leggy perennials—certainly not the landscape that inspires imagination. Today, a veritable oasis of organic produce encourages children, teachers, and parents to learn more about food, nature, and healthy eating.

The mission of the Edible Schoolyard is unique, and aims to "create and sustain an organic garden and landscape that is wholly integrated into the school's curriculum, culture and food program. ESY involves students in all aspects of farming the garden and preparing, serving and eating food as a means of awakening their senses and encouraging awareness and appreciation of the transformative values of nourishment, community and stewardship of the land."[16] After a quick walk through the facility, it is clear that the goals are being met. The garden is planted with seasonal produce, herbs, berries, and fruit trees. There is also a tool shed, seed propagation table, chicken coop, and a pizza oven.

The Edible Schoolyard is part of the curriculum for all students at King Middle School. In the fall, sixth graders—as part of their math and science curriculum—work in the garden while seventh graders in the humanities and social science classes start in the kitchen. Come spring, the classes trade places. The eighth graders use the garden year-round for science classes or specialized projects. When finished with the curriculum, the students will have gained a complete seed-to-table experience, which begins by preparing and seeding the planting beds and concludes with a sit-down meal at the table, complete with flowers from the garden. (And something parents will find most amazing, the children even participate in the cleanup!) Throughout the school year, the program exposes children to food production, ecology, and nutrition, and fosters an appreciation of meaningful work, and of fresh and natural food.

The Edible Schoolyard program at King Middle School has become so admired that the garden is visited by more than 1,000 people each year, from all over the world. Educators, healthcare professionals—even legislators—come to learn how the seeds of this program could be planted in their communities. This unique program has spawned hundreds of kitchen and garden programs throughout the world. Because of its comprehensive curriculum and the important life lessons that are taught, the Edible School-yard is arguably the benchmark by which any food education program is measured, whether it is aimed at children or adults.

Obviously, a full-fledged edible schoolyard on the scale of King Middle School is a massive undertaking. But even one small garden plot can offer profound lessons to children (and parents) on food. Setting aside an hour to plant seeds, and a few minutes each week to water, weed, and study how food evolves in a patch of dirt, can have an immensely positive impact on even the youngest grade-school children.

Outside my daughter's kindergarten class in northern California, there was talk one day between some of the parents about establishing a small garden plot. Food is important in this region, and many parents have urged the school to adopt a healthier attitude toward food. But as with any project, there were hurdles to clear.

Our problem wasn't the usual one when trying to start a garden: infrastructure. We had water. We also had a tool shed. In fact, we even had a raised garden box filled with soil. What we didn't have was gumption. The teacher wasn't enthused about incorporating gardening into the school curriculum, but offered, "If this is something parents wish to do, I will support you guys in your efforts."

So another parent and I purchased some seeds and seedlings, and then took an hour out of our day and held a gardening work-shop for the kids. We planted fun stuff we thought kids would enjoy growing, like rainbow chard; yellow, red, and purple carrots; orange cauliflower; red radishes; and green peas. We planted stuff that was fun to touch and smell, like sage. We planted stevia, because we thought kids would be amazed that something green and leafy could taste like candy. And we even planted the strange:

Brussels sprouts. The kids learned about food and where it comes from. They also learned about roots and flowers and leaves and dirt. And they had a blast.

The two of us watered the box regularly, and managed the weeds and bugs. But what had sprouted was more than we could have hoped for. When the seedlings emerged, so did the teacher's enthusiasm for the garden. She started helping out with the watering. She helped kids pick radishes, and she even took handfuls of chard home to her family on occasion. Many of the other parents became intrigued with the garden as well, as they often gathered around the plot and ogled the growing vegetables while they waited for their kids to get out of school. The amount of food the garden yielded was modest. But the joy it brought kids and parents, and the interest in fresh vegetables that the garden sparked, was immeasurable.

Gathering parents, teachers, and schoolchildren together to plant a garden helps us all regain that once strong agrarian knowledge.

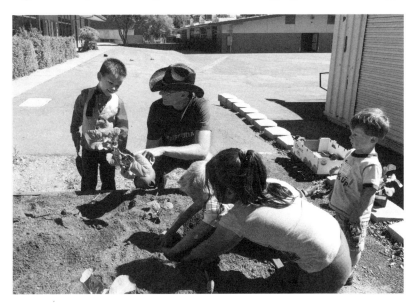

The author and kindergarten children plant vegetables in a garden outside the classroom. He has dubbed the group the KinderGardeners.

Likewise, the myriad programs, events, demonstrations, teaching gardens, and displays created by food advocacy groups, motivated citizens, and municipalities illustrate creative strategies to increase food literacy in North America. The benefits of being food literate are that we gain an appreciation for food, its diversity, and all the places and methods of its production. These educational efforts foster nutritional, social, and environmental awareness, and are part and parcel of any successful system of public produce.

Public officials should play an active role in educating citizens about healthier food choices, but they needn't create a custom-tailored food curriculum. Models to emulate are everywhere. Great ideas abound on the Internet. Citizens throughout the community are willing to help. All it takes is a few folks with a willingness to gather information and a passion to spread knowledge throughout the community. Once the information is assembled and disseminated, we can be assured of a healthier, food-savvy society.

Conclusion

Community Health
and Prosperity

Public space is arguably every city's greatest, most abundant physical resource. The multitude of streets, parks, squares, and plazas are where people from all walks of life come together to socialize with familiar faces, make new acquaintances, and simply revel in one another's company. Public space thus builds community, and because this is where different people share different ideas, public space also helps sow the seeds of democracy. In these ways, public space nourishes our soul. But might these places nourish our body as well?

Growing food in public space is not a new idea, but one that is timely and worth revisiting. From the late nineteenth century to the mid-twentieth, government had asked city dwellers to help mitigate economic and social distress through urban agriculture on public land. The efforts from the victory garden campaign, perhaps the most successful of the various government-sponsored public agriculture efforts, were staggering. By 1944, there were an estimated twenty million victory gardens yielding eight million tons of produce, collectively providing 40 percent of the nation's vegetable supply.[1]

More than food, however, victory gardens and their earlier urban farming counterparts promoted self-reliance, self-respect, and economic independence, providing financial, physical, and spiritual well-being. And because these forms of public produce were established in many neighborhoods, involving many neighbors, they helped build and nurture community, as well. Some cities, like Boston, have never lost sight of the value of these earlier programs of urban food production. Indeed, the seven-acre Fenway Victory Gardens, a link in the city's famed Emerald Necklace of public parks, has been continuously cultivated since 1942. Other cities are rediscovering the value of victory gardens. In 2008, the City of San Francisco funded a victory garden pilot program that established a 10,000-square-foot edible garden right in front of City Hall—the same spot where the city had its original victory garden sixty-five years earlier. Seeking to increase local food security and decrease the food miles associated with the average American meal, San Francisco's program equates "victory" to fewer carbon dioxide emissions, self-reliance, seasonal growing and eating, community action, and most notably, independence from corporate food systems.[2]

San Francisco's victory garden program illustrates the broad goals of community food production, and the inherent environmental and societal benefits of growing food on public land. In fact, the goals of the original victory garden campaign of World War II were also broad, affecting not just food security, but individual economic assistance as well as family morale. During a National Defense Gardening Conference, held on December 19, 1941, the secretary of agriculture and the director of the US Office of Defense, Health, and Welfare Services articulated the far-reaching aims of the victory garden campaign:

Increase the production and consumption of fresh vegetables and fruits by more and better home, school, and community gardens, to the end that we become a stronger and healthier nation.

Encourage the proper storage and preservation of the surplus from such gardens for distribution and use by families producing it, local school lunches, welfare agencies, and for local emergency food needs.

Enable families and institutions to save on the cost of vegetables and to apply this saving to other necessary foods which must be purchased.

Provide, through the medium of community gardens, an opportunity for gardening by urban dwellers and others who lack suitable home garden facilities.

Maintain and improve the morale and spiritual well-being of the individual, family and nation.[3]

The goals for victory gardens then are just as relevant as those of public produce today. There are some differences in organization and operation, however. For one, the big push for urban food security during the victory garden campaign came from Washington. Whereas the federal government provided encouragement and guidance, municipal government—and its local citizens—provided action. For future urban food-producing endeavors, municipal government will likely have to provide both impetus and implementation. Certainly, if central government today adopted a food attitude similar to that exhibited during World War II, it would be welcome. Today's federal government, with its now sixty-year favor of centralized, industrial agriculture, seems unlikely to change their attitude soon.

Even if that attitude does change, it may not be as effective as local-government policy. As Mark Winne argues, "Democracy works best when it's closest to the people. That is why we can expect city hall to act faster than the state capitol, which in turn tends to respond to its people before Washington, DC. The farther away the decision makers are from those whose lives are affected by their decisions, the slower will be the change that occurs."⁴

Public produce will also need to be regarded with more permanence than the earlier food security programs. The potato patches, liberty gardens, depression relief gardens, and victory gardens were all ephemeral (Boston's Fenway Victory Gardens excluded). They existed within a finite time of economic and social distress, and promptly vanished once prosperity rebounded.

Though the success of victory gardens provoked many to fight for their continuance, the end of the war and the transition to an industrial system of agriculture left the government—and the general public—without desire to maintain the prolific and abundant urban gardens. While the exploding middle class and higher socioeconomic strata enjoyed benefits from the industrial agriculture boom, the inner-city poor were still left without an adequate supply of food. As suburbs consumed farmland outside the cities, and supermarkets and grocery stores followed the mass emigration of the post-war population, food problems were exacerbated for inner-city residents. Today, however, food insecurity is threatening more than the urban poor. Folks across all socioeconomic standings are feeling those hunger pangs that our grandparents and great-grandparents felt last century. But this time, in the face of climate change and a shrinking oil supply, we will require community food-producing activities with longevity. History has taught us that we can no longer believe that community health and prosperity lie in a centralized, corporate system of food production. Indeed, it is precisely this system that has contributed to the food crisis we currently face. If allowed to continue, and if history of other fallen nations is any indicator, we may lose any chance of regaining economic prosperity.

Eric Schlosser, in his best-selling book *Fast Food Nation*, drew frightening parallels between our current system of agriculture and that of the former Soviet Union:

Throughout the Cold War, America's decentralized system of agriculture, relying upon millions of independent producers, was depicted as the most productive system in the world, as proof of capitalism's inherent superiority. The perennial crop failures in the Soviet Union were attributed to a highly centralized system run by distant bureaucrats. Today the handful of agribusiness firms that dominate American food production are championing another centralized system of production, one in which livestock and farmland are viewed purely as commodities, farmers are reduced to the status of employees, and crop decisions are made by executives far away from the fields.[5]

Recently, the United States witnessed the vulnerability of such a centralized system. When storms flooded the corn fields of Iowa in June 2008, inundating 1.3 million acres of that cropland, amidst rising fuel prices and the divergence of corn from food to biofuel, prices for beef, pork, poultry, eggs, milk, and cheese soared not only across the country, but throughout the world. Our reliance on oil to produce corn in Iowa, and corn to produce ethanol to combat the high price of oil, and the weather anomalies and climate change that have resulted from decades of burning both oil and ethanol, has locked us into an unsustainable cyclone that, if left to perpetuate, will decimate our food supply. The complex interplay between corn, oil, climate change, and the price and availability of food today illustrates an urgency to return to a more decentralized system of agriculture, closer to, and within, our cities, where the majority of Americans are now living. A network of public produce, grown on underutilized public land using plentiful and readily available sunshine, can help decentralize our system of agriculture and increase food security.

Critics, I expect, will contend that serious food production requires land—lots of land—and the skill, knowledge, and machinery necessary to produce the quantities of food citizens demand. The victory garden effort proves otherwise. Regardless, public produce is not meant to annihilate the current food machine, or undermine the relationships that communities are building with smaller, regional farms. My hunch is that there will always be a need for some form of corporate industrial agriculture (though it will have to be scaled back), and there will always be a desire to have independent family farms within a couple hours drive of the city. Public produce merely offers yet another choice, and there is certainly room for all. That is what cities have always been, and should continue to be, about: providing choice. But the fact remains that the vast majority of agricultural land does not produce food to feed us directly. Rather, the overwhelming majority of agricultural land is used to produce feed for livestock, or else it is used in the manufacturing of processed foods, such as high-fructose corn syrup, partially hydrogenated fats, and enriched grain flours that find their way into the myriad soft drinks, cereals, snack foods, and baked goods that currently represent staples in the American diet.

Farmers' markets have recently exploded in popularity and provide healthful, much-needed dietary alternatives to the big food-producing corporations. While the quality of what is offered at farmers' markets is often better than what is found at supermarkets, this lower yield and higher quality come at a price. Community-supported agriculture (CSA) groups can offer a cheaper alternative, but choice is limited. A member of any such group only receives produce that his or her CSA grows. This is especially disappointing for ethnic families, who seek the more "exotic" produce items for their traditional cuisines. And CSAs generally do not give you the opportunity to specify how much of a particular produce item you want (or may need) each week; you get what you get. While CSAs and farmers' markets can add variety and help supplement what we buy at the grocery store, there is still need for additional, cost-effective produce choices, especially for those who cannot afford the alternatives. This is where municipalities can help.

As civil servants, municipal officials need to implement programs and policies that meet the needs and desires of their citizens, and access to healthy food has been a need within urban communities for decades. While there have been attempts at urban food production since the victory garden campaign, these attempts have failed, principally because of the lack of initiative and support from the community leaders and policy makers.

During the 1996 American Community Gardening Association conference, Laura Lawson brought up the intractable concerns of sustaining urban gardening longevity. In her book *City Bountiful*, Lawson writes, "Once we put aside our pictures of happy children and inspirational stories, we found that we were all struggling with similar concerns. Everyone was committed to the idea of gardening as a resource to serve the social, environmental, and economic needs of urban, low-income communities, but everyone also felt pressured by insecure land tenure, competitive funding, staff burnout, and the need to sustain community-based leadership."[6] These issues, which have persisted for decades with community gardens, will likely continue with any public food-growing effort, unless local government adopts a proactive attitude and takes a hands-on approach to fresh-produce production. Securing land, allocating funds, and dedicating municipal staff to the issues of public produce can help ensure community food security. And it goes beyond meeting the food needs of the poor. In addition to assisting low-income communities that currently have limited access to fresh produce, public produce can aid middle-class Americans, who are increasingly discovering that farmers' market produce is beyond their financial reach. As well, it can meet the demands of the upper class, who increasingly insist that the food they consume—be it in their homes or in posh restaurants—be locally grown. And public produce can aid all folks who have simply grown tired of conventional agriculture and desire a little glimpse of the agrarian life that this land of opportunity was founded upon.

Aside from obvious economic and environmental benefits of public produce, there are intrinsic civic benefits to be gleaned as well. Municipal government, as it works toward that ultimate goal of building healthful and prosperous communities, should embrace the social benefits of public produce as being equally important as the environmental and economic ones. As Luc Mougeot contends, "Urban agriculture is not the total solution to issues facing the future of cities, but it is an essential part of any program to make those cities more livable, and to improve the lives of city dwellers."[7]

One societal characteristic of urban agriculture that differs from conventional agriculture is the democratization of community-based food production. Unless food consumers are part of the family corporations of industrial agriculture, or sit on the boards of the larger, public corporations, they have little voice in food choice. Voting with one's pocketbook is not entirely rational when it comes to food, as it often is with other retail endeavors. People have to eat. If the choice is between supermarket produce that they may be able to afford versus farmers' market produce which is certainly out of their financial reach, there is truly no choice. Such purchasing patterns erroneously suggest that people "prefer" supermarket produce, because that is what the majority of people buy.

Public produce, on the other hand, gives consumers a significant voice in food production. Because it is on public land, the public has a direct say in how that land is managed, either through the democratic process of electing leaders (mayors and members of the council), lobbying those already elected about food policies, or merely relating concerns to the stewards of those lands (municipal staff members or community volunteers, for example)—those they see every day on their way to work, school, or places of commerce, recreation, or worship. And, not to forget, these municipal land stewards—city staff that grow the produce, and maintain the garden plots—are themselves members of the community.

A system of public produce thus yields a new type of member in the community—one the late Thomas Lyson called a "food citizen." The idea is that public produce, a form of food production that fits within Lyson's definition of *civic agriculture*, gives citizens a voice that is currently muted in our conventional food-supply system. Lyson reasoned:

> Civic agriculture flourishes in a democratic environment. Problem solving around the social, economic, and environmental issues related to agriculture and food requires that all citizens have a say in how the agriculture and food system is organized. Indeed, citizen participation in agriculture and food-related organizations and associations is a cornerstone of civic agriculture. Through active engagement in the food system, civic agriculture has the potential to transform individuals from passive consumers into active food citizens. A food citizen is someone who has not only a stake but also a voice in how and where his or her food is produced, processed, and sold.
>
> The free-market neoclassical system of conventional agriculture, on the other hand, does not necessarily benefit from democracy and, in fact, may be constrained by the politics put into place through democratic actions of citizens.[8]

Civic agriculture, as Lyson contended, holds value to everyone in the community. One group that society increasingly finds difficult to engage is teenagers. After Mark Winne started the Natick Community Farm in Massachusetts in 1975, he and his colleagues had found that the farm had an unexpected value for teenagers, especially at-risk youth. Principally, community farming, as Winne discovered, provides a positive outlook for these youngsters. He noted, "It has . . . become increasingly important that the town's young people have an alternative frame of reference that doesn't include the local mall and that gives them a respite from an economic system that treats them as if they are only consumers-in-training." The ultimate value, Winne realized, was that these urban agriculture endeavors "have amply demonstrated that life offers a richer menu of choices."[9]

If San Francisco is any indication, this richer menu of choice even has value for society's seemingly incorrigible. Similar to Winne's observations that urban agriculture gives teenagers an alternative frame of reference that doesn't include the typical teen hangouts, urban agriculture offers offenders in San Francisco an alternative frame of reference from the troubled streets of their community. Former inmates raise organic vegetables, such as radishes, kale, chard, and broccoli—as well as many varieties of fruits—on land owned by the San Francisco City and County jail. The Garden Project, the moniker of this unique urban agriculture program, aims to prevent crime and reduce recidivism. And it has proved quite successful. San Francisco County sheriff Mike Hennessey notes, "The Garden Project is a tremendously effective crime-prevention program. It not only helps individuals rebuild their lives, but recidivism studies we've conducted also show that while 55 percent of our prisoners are rearrested within a year, those who go through The Garden Project have a recidivism rate of 24 percent, and that's after two years."[10]

Crack dealers, hookers, assailants, and scores of at-risk youth have gone on the straight and narrow simply from growing organic food. Outside this municipal garden, the same streets are still wracked with crime, homelessness, drugs, and prostitution. But through gardening, these former offenders find solace, and learn about hope. *New York Times* reporter Jane Gross, who covered The Garden Project many years ago, poetically relayed the deeper meaning of growing organic produce. Gross reflects that the leeks, raspberries, and potatoes that flourish in the jailhouse garden "are not merely fruits and vegetables. Rather they are metaphors for what went wrong in a prisoner's troubled past, lessons about how to live a healthy and honorable life, and proof that love and work make a garden flourish." Gross even saw the value that pulling weeds can have on recovering from such a troubled past. "The simple process of weeding is a good place to start re-examining a life gone wrong. The weeds are whatever got in the way: smoking crack or whoring or stealing. Once they are gone, no longer leaching water and nutrients from all that grows around them, the vegetables and fruits thrive."[11]

Mark Winne believes that "the power of community gardening and other similarly organized small-scale farming efforts in nontraditional areas such as urban America is not found so much in the rate of return to the food supply but in the rate of return to society."[12] When criminals are rehabilitated, the rate of return to society is extremely high. These one-time public offenders now help the people they used to hurt. The food that is produced by The Garden Project used to be sold to many tony restaurants in the San Francisco Bay Area. Today, the produce has a higher calling; it is used to feed the city's many elderly and poor families. The one-time criminals growing this food earn a modest income, which helps them get by from day to day. What has greater value to them, and to society, are the life lessons they learn, which yield positive returns beyond their immediate future.

Imagine the comprehensive network of public produce that could result if one municipality aggregated all of the individual urban agriculture efforts undertaken in other communities: the San Francisco sheriff who helps organize a rehabilitation garden for former offenders in his community; the mayor in Chicago who orders a honeybee colony on the roof of City Hall; the city planner in Provo who grows vegetables outside his City Hall office; the urban foresters in Davenport and Calgary who plant fruit trees in neighborhood parks; the pair of students who lobbied Seattle's Public Utilities to plant a food forest on their underutilized land; the councilmember in Worthington who advocates for transitional gardens to help feed the less fortunate; the legislators in Montpelier who plant vegetables as part of an ornamental landscape outside the State House; the Los Angeles organization Fallen Fruit that publishes maps alerting people to the whereabouts of publicly accessible fruit in the city, and when it is ready to harvest; and the restaurant staff in Berkeley who are willing to trade meals for Meyer lemons. All of these seemingly disparate local agricultural and food-production efforts, when coalesced into one program that provides assistance to the individual while bettering the community, comprise a model worth creating, and subsequently emulating.

There has been a call by some of our greatest food advocates and thinkers—like Eric Schlosser, Marion Nestle, Michael Pollan, and Alice Waters—for a change in federal government policy toward food and food production. The first step toward policy reform, many argue, must come from the American president himself. Michael Pollan contends there is tremendous "power of the example you set in the White House. If what's needed is a change of culture in America's thinking about food, then how America's first household organizes its eating will set the national tone, focusing the light of public attention on the issue and communicating a simple set of values that guide Americans toward sun-based foods and away from eating oil."[13]

And the White House responded. During the Obama administration, 1,100 square feet of South Lawn sod was turned into an organic vegetable garden. The principal reason for the garden, according to First Lady Michelle Obama, was "to educate children about healthful, locally grown fruit and vegetables at a time when obesity and diabetes have become a national concern."[14] Pollan was right; the modest garden has sent a symbolic message to families throughout the country that it is time to reassess what we eat and how we produce it.

While the White House vegetable garden is inspiring, the problem is still the elephant on the dinner plate: our corporately controlled, centralized system of agriculture. The presidential veggie patch sends a loud and laudable message to families who have both land and leisure to grow their own food. But these initiatives don't do much to modify behavior of the current beast, by rethinking how we can deliver fresh fruit and vegetables to citizens who need it most—those who do not have the time, space, ability, or financial wherewithal to secure it for themselves. The next evolution of public agriculture should be toward healthful, organic, local food of the people, by the people, and for the people, to paraphrase Abraham Lincoln. The First Family's garden is an ennobling gesture, but urban agriculture needs to do more by serving more.

The time has come for a "re-org" of our centralized food production system. Access to healthful food should not be a privilege, but a fundamental right. The current agricultural production methods no longer seem ideal for much of our population. As the demand—and need—for affordable, locally produced food rises, it is becoming abundantly clear from the success stories to date that the most effective food policies lie not within a central government body, but within a local one. If daily access to safe, nutritious, culturally acceptable produce, at little to no cost, is necessary to improve the wealth and health of city dwellers, then city government will need to lead the charge.

Because, in the very near future, the strength of our country may be determined by the ability of our communities to feed themselves.

Acknowledgments

As an urban designer, I typically frame my thoughts around cities. It's a handicap at times, but for the purpose of thanking the numerous individuals who assisted with this book, it's the best way to organize my gratitude.

The journey for this new edition of *Public Produce* began in Washington, DC. It's not often an author gets an opportunity to inject new life into a five-year-old book. Or the chance to completely revise it, improving both content and style. I have Courtney Lix at Island Press to thank for that. In fact, I have Courtney to thank for just about every improvement to *Public Produce*. Her insights, editorial prowess, and incredible patience make her about the best editor in the literate universe. And she has become a dear friend in the process. Thank you, Courtney.

Actually, every accolade and achievement I have garnered through writing I owe to the staff at Island Press. Heather Boyer was my first editorial partner, and she has been involved in each of my three books going back to 2007. It was because of Heather's tireless championing of this work to her editorial board that *Public Produce* was published. If you love the book, you too owe Heather a heartfelt "Thank you!"

Jaime Jennings is Island Press's energetic publicist and a better promoter of my work than I am. Sharis Simonian, Meghan Bartels, Angela Osborn, Jason Leppig, Maureen Gately, and Chuck Savitt have all been extremely supportive and helpful, and I owe you all a tremendous debt of gratitude.

In Davenport, Iowa, I wish to give hearty thanks to Tom Flaherty. Before I wrote the first edition of this book, public produce was a fantasy in my head. Tom showed me it could be a reality. Indeed, if it weren't for Tom's inspiring efforts—growing all those tomatoes, corn, beans, and peppers outside his downtown office window for anyone to harvest—this book would have never been written. I also wish to thank former Horticulture Manager Susan Anderson and City Arborist Chris Johnson, both of whom inspired me with their innovative and sensitive manner of stewarding municipal land.

Just a few miles west, thanks goes to Teva Dawson in Des Moines for her assistance with the first edition of this book and for follow-up advice on this edition. Callie Le'au Cartwright manages the City of Des Moines' community garden program and was very generous with her time, answering my many questions.

Seattle is filled with inspiring folks bent on improving food security in their community. Trudi Inslee drove me all over her city, introducing me to many of these food pioneers. She also facilitated radio and newspaper interviews and public speaking engagements, so that I could share this idea of produce by the people, for the people.

Gail Savina of Seattle's City Fruit was especially enlightening with regard to the economics of public produce. And she proved to be an excellent soundboard for my arguments, correcting me when I erred in my logic. Jacqueline Cramer and Glenn Herlihy, code-signers of the Beacon Food Forest, shared passionate insights into the hows, whats, and whys of their project. I learned a lot from this pioneering duo, and I thank you both for your tutelage.

Whenever I speak on the topic of public produce, the highlight of my talk is Provo, Utah. The audience just loves Nathan Murray's annual endeavor to turn Provo City Hall into a public vegetable patch. Nathan has been an excellent mentor over the last five years, and his inspiring efforts help folks see the inherent joy in growing food for anyone to harvest.

Carl Etnier and Glenn Scherer in Montpelier, Vermont, allowed me to promote *Public Produce* through radio and newspaper editorials. And their involvement in transforming the State House lawn into an ornamental *and* edible landscape opened my eyes to the latent beauty of vegetables. Patricia Foster and Melissa Grim from the City of Baltimore were kind to answer questions about their community's City Hall vegetable garden. Worthington, Ohio councilman Doug Smith cut short his family dinner one evening to give me a tour of the transitional gardens in his city. And Michael Thompson—beekeeper extraordinaire—provided the history of the City of Chicago's municipal apiaries.

I wish to detour north to thank the many inspiring individuals implementing public produce in Canada. Jill-Anne Spence provided fantastic information on the City of Calgary's Community Orchard Project, while Daphne Powell, a planner with the City of Nelson, walked me through her community's zoning laws.

But it is in Kamloops, British Columbia, where I owe my deepest international gratitude. Laura Kalina, Elaine Sedgman, and Kendra Besanger continue to inspire me. Their tireless promotion of public produce (both the concept and my book) is humbling. But it is what they taught me that leaves me indebted to this trio. Better than anyone else in North America, Laura, Elaine, and Kendra taught me how to educate a community about food and food security. Their lessons were always joyful and salubrious. All three are gifted mentors with boundless passion. Thank you, thank you, thank you.

Back home, Stacie Pierce, pastry chef at Berkeley's famed Chez Panisse, took much-appreciated time from her busy schedule to talk with me about the evolving food and foraging philosophy in the San Francisco Bay Area. She is obviously passionate about cuisine, culture, and the environment, and her commitment to locally sourced food is inspiring.

This project could not have been completed without the broad aid and comfort of family. Mary and Dave Nordahl, and Donna and Ken Jensen provided shelter, food, transportation, and welcomed childcare. We disrupted their lifestyles and living arrangements for months during the first edition of this book and again during this revision. But I hope the intimate time spent with their grandchildren was just compensation.

Many thanks to my brother, Derek Nordahl, and my "siblings-in-law": Todd Jensen, Greg and Heather McAvoy-Jensen, and Viviana Nordahl. Derek was very helpful—on short notice—with illustrations for the book. Todd provided ample work space, provocative conversation, excellent food, and fine drink (the latter of which stimulated even more provocative conversation). Greg provided needed books for reference, as well as relevant online articles. His wife, Heather, provided considerate support and encouragement, both to me and, more important, to my wife. Vivi kept me abreast of all the food headlines and happenings in the Bay Area. She forwarded many articles related to urban agriculture, and was as close to a graduate student researcher that an author outside of academe could hope to have.

Finally, I would like to express my most earnest gratitude to my wife, for her unconditional love, support, and enduring friendship. She is truly my biggest champion, and my greatest source of inspiration. Thank you, Lara.

Notes

Introduction

1. These are statistics provided by Ron Finley. The US Department of Agriculture (USDA) estimates 23.5 million Americans live in a food desert. Regardless of whose numbers you believe, we have a serious food problem in America.

2. All quotes and statistics, unless otherwise noted, taken from Ron Finley, "A Guerilla Gardener in South Central LA," *TED2013 Talks*, February 2013, http://www.ted.com/talks/ron_finley_a_guerilla_gardener_in_south_central_la.html (last accessed January 23, 2014).

3. Thomas A. Lyson, *Civic Agriculture: Reconnecting Farm, Food, and Community* (Lebanon, NH: University Press of New England, 2004), 21.

4. In 2008, Wendy's launched an ad campaign that sought to distinguish its menu items from fast food. Though its menu still heavily comprised fried hamburgers, French fries, chicken nuggets, soft drinks, and shakes, the tagline that concluded each commercial was, "It's waaaay better than fast food. It's Wendy's."

5. Kent Garber, "At Last, Some Respect for Fruits and Veggies," *U.S. News & World Report*, March 13, 2008, Nation section.

6. Holly Hill, "Food Miles and Marketing," National Sustainable Agriculture Information Service, http://attra.ncat.org/attra-pub/foodmiles.html (last accessed June 19, 2014).

7. Lauren Shepherd, "McDonald's 1Q Profit Rises Nearly 4 Percent," *The Huffington Post,* April 22, 2009, http://www.huffingtonpost.com/2009/04/22/mcdonalds-profit-rises-ne_n_189923.html (last accessed May 9, 2009).

8. Susan Anderson, in an e-mail message to the author, July 8, 2008.

9. Lyson, 62–64.

10. Farmers' markets statistics are from the USDA Agricultural Marketing Service, as of the first week of August, 2013, http://www.ams.usda.gov/AMSv1.0/farmersmarkets (last accessed January 24, 2014). The CSA statistics are from Steven McFadden, "Unraveling the CSA Conundrum," *The Call of the Land* blog (and book), http://thecalloftheland.wordpress

.com/2012/01/09/unraveling-the-csa-number-conundrum/ (last accessed April 2, 2014).

11. The Oxford University Press anointed "locavore" the 2007 Word of the Year, http://blog.oup.com/2007/11/locavore/ (last accessed November 1, 2008).

12. Anderson, 2008.

Chapter 1

1. Governor Edmund G. Brown in a press conference delivered January 17, 2014.

2. Bryan Walsh, "Hundred Years of Dry: How California's Drought Could Get Much, Much Worse," *Time*, January 23, 2014, http://time.com/1986/hundred-years-of-dry-how-californias-drought-could-get-much-much-worse/ (last accessed June 19, 2014).

3. Governor Edmund G. Brown in his annual State of the State address, January 22, 2014. The full transcript of the address can be seen here: http://www.turnto23.com/news/local-news/watch-live-gov-jerry-brown-delivers-state-of-the-state-address (last accessed January 25, 2014).

4. California Agriculture Statistics Overview 2012–2013, http://www.cdfa.ca.gov/statistics/ (last accessed January 25, 2014).

5. Eric Schlosser, *Fast Food Nation* (New York: Perennial, 2002), 266.

6. Sophie Wenzlau, "Global Food Prices Continue to Rise," *Worldwatch Institute*, April 11, 2013: http://www.worldwatch.org/global-food-prices-continue-rise-0 (last accessed January 25, 2014).

7. Kent Garber, "Midwest Floods Ruin Crops," *U.S. News & World Report*, June 18, 2008, http://www.usnews.com/news/national/articles/2008/06/18/midwest-floods-ruin-crops (last accessed January 25, 2014).

8. Woody Barth, "The Real Cause of Rising Food Prices," *The Hill*, June 20, 2013, http://thehill.com/blogs/congress-blog/economy-a-budget/306313-the-real-cause-of-rising-food-prices (last accessed January 25, 2014).

9. Michael Pollan, "Farmer in Chief," *New York Times Magazine*, October 12, 2008, New York edition, MM62.

10. James Howard Kunstler, *The Long Emergency: Surviving the End of Oil, Climate Change, and Other Converging Catastrophes of the Twenty-First Century* (New York: Grove Press, 2005), 239.

11. Laura J. Lawson, *City Bountiful* (Berkeley: University of California Press, 2005), 171.

12. Ibid., 115.

13. Juanita Kakalec, in a conversation with the author, March 23, 2008.

14. Daniel Solomon, *Global City Blues* (Washington, DC: Island Press, 2003), 17.

15. Mark Winne, *Closing the Food Gap: Resetting the Table in the Land of Plenty.* (Boston: Beacon Press, 2008).

16. Rich Pirog et al., *Food, Fuel, and Freeways: An Iowa perspective on how far food travels, fuel usage, and greenhouse gas emissions* (Ames, IA: Leopold Center for Sustainable Agriculture, Iowa State University, 2001). An interesting graphic associated with the report, which illustrates how far selected produce varieties travel by truck to reach a terminal market in Chicago, can be viewed at http://www.leopold.iastate.edu/pubs/staff/ppp/produce_chart.html (last accessed May 10, 2009).

17. Sue Weaver, "Origins of the Orchard," *Orcharding* 8 (2008): 8.

18. Pirog, 6.

19. Data on Iowa's commodity crops and cash receipts were obtained from the US Department of Agriculture's Economic Research Service. Data sets for all commodities by state can be obtained from http://www.ers.usda.gov/data-products/farm-income-and-wealth-statistics/annual-cash-receipts-by-commodity.aspx#Pd0ace6f4615d4822a32fe0d23beef6be_2_22iT0T0R0x15 (last accessed April 2, 2014).

20. For more information about the FDA's Produce Safety Action Plan, visit http://www.fda.gov/Food/FoodborneIllnessContaminants/BuyStoreServeSafeFood/ucm2006739.htm (last accessed April 2, 2014).

21. Center for Food Safety and Applied Nutrition, "Lettuce Safety Initiative," US Food and Drug Administration (August 23, 2006), http://www.fda.gov/Food/FoodborneIllnessContaminants/BuyStoreServeSafeFood/ucm115906.htm (last accessed April 2, 2014).

22. For a documented history of the *E. coli* outbreak in spinach, including state-by-state statistics, visit the CDC website, http://www.cdc.gov/ecoli/2006/september/updates/ (last accessed May 10, 2009).

23. US Food and Drug Administration/Center for Food Safety and Applied Nutrition, "Leafy Greens Safety Initiative—2nd year," October 4, 2007, http://www.fda.gov/Food/FoodborneIllnessContaminants/BuyStoreServeSafeFood/ucm115898.htm (last accessed April 2, 2014).

24. Information on the outbreak of *Salmonella saintpaul*-tainted peppers, including state-by-state statistics for this particular outbreak, can be found on the CDC web site, http://www.cdc.gov/salmonella/saintpaul/jalapeno/ (last accessed May 10, 2009).

25. Information on the outbreak of *Salmonella typhimurium*, including state-by-state statistics for this serotype, can be found on the CDC

website, http://www.cdc.gov/salmonella/typhimurium/update.html (last accessed May 10, 2009).

26. Ricardo Alonso-Zaldivar, "Private Inspections of Food Companies Seen as Weak," Associated Press, March 20, 2009, http://www.foxnews .com/printer_friendly_wires/2009Mar20/0,4675,SalmonellaOutbreak ,00.htm (last accessed April 2, 2014).

27. Ricardo Alonso-Zaldivar and Brett J. Blackledge, "Stewart Parnell, Peanut Corp Owner, Refuses to Testify to Congress in Salmonella Hearing," Associated Press, February 11, 2009, http://www.huffingtonpost .com/2009/02/11/stewart-parnell-peanut-co_n_166058.html (last accessed May 10, 2009).

28. Centers for Disease Control and Prevention, "Multistate Outbreak of Shiga Toxin-producing *Escherichia coli* O26 Infections Linked to Raw Clover Sprouts at Jimmy John's Restaurants (Final Update)," April 3, 2012, http://www.cdc.gov/ecoli/2012/o26-02-12/index.html (last accessed January 25, 2014).

29. Centers for Disease Control and Prevention, "Salmonella," http:// www.cdc.gov/salmonella/outbreaks.html (last accessed January 25, 2014).

30. Results from the AP-Ipsos poll were gleaned from Ricardo Alonso-Zaldivar, "Food Safety Worries Change Buying Habits," ABC News, July 18, 2008, http://usatoday30.usatoday.com/news/nation/2008-07-18-353 1246574_x.htm (last accessed April 2, 2014).

31. Ibid.

32. Marion Nestle, in an e-mail exchange with the author, October 15, 2008.

33. Pollan, "Farmer in Chief."

34. Amanda Gardner, "FDA Expands Tomato Warning Nationwide," HealthDayNews, June 10, 2008, http://www.healthday.com/Article.asp ?AID=616391 (last accessed November 28, 2008).

35. Centers for Disease Control and Prevention, "Outbreak of Salmonella Serotype Saintpaul Infections Associated with Multiple Raw Produce Items—United States, 2008," *Morbidity and Mortality Weekly Report* 57, no. 34 (August 29, 2008), 929–34.

36. Centers for Disease Control and Prevention/Division of Foodborne, Bacterial and Mycotic Diseases, "Salmonellosis," http://www.cdc .gov/salmonella/ (last accessed April 2, 2014).

37. World Health Organization, *Guidelines for the Safe Use of Wastewater, Excreta and Greywater*, vol. 4 of *Excreta and Greywater Use in*

Agriculture (Geneva: WHO Press, 2006), http://www.who.int/water
_sanitation_health/wastewater/gsuweg4/en/.

38. Marion Nestle, *Safe Food: Bacteria, Biotechnology, and Bioterrorism*
(Berkeley: University of California Press, 2003), 59.

39. Ibid.

40. As reported in Pollan, "Farmer in Chief."

41. Ibid.

42. Kristin Collins, "Grower Settles with Limbless Child," *News & Observer* (Raleigh, NC), March 25, 2008, B1.

43. Information regarding lead contamination in soil and remediation strategies, including specific quotes, was gleaned from Carl J. Rosen, "Lead in the Home Garden and Urban Soil Environment," University of Minnesota Extension, 2002, http://www.extension.umn.edu/distribution
/horticulture/DG2543.html (last accessed January 29, 2009).

44. Pollan, "Farmer in Chief."

Chapter 2

1. Colin Beavan, "The No Impact Experiment," *The No Impact Man Blog*, entry posted February 21, 2007, http://noimpactman.typepad.com
/blog/2007/02/the_no_impact_e.html (last accessed February 3, 2014).

2. Colin Beaven, "Like Falling Off a Log," *The No Impact Man Blog*, entry posted March 21, 2008, http://noimpactman.typepad.com/blog/2008/03
/like-falling-of.html (last accessed February 3, 2014).

3. Michael Pollan, *The Omnivore's Dilemma: A Natural History of Four Meals* (New York: Penguin, 2006), 100–108.

4. Michael Pollan, *In Defense of Food: An Eater's Manifesto* (New York: Penguin , 2008), 158.

5. Nutrition information for peaches obtained from, Frances Sizer and Eleanor Whitney, *Nutrition: Concepts and Controversies,* 6th ed. (Minneapolis/St. Paul: West Publishing, 1994), A-20. Nutrition information for McDonald's double cheeseburger and other menu items available at: http://www.mcdonalds.com/us/en/food/full_menu/sandwiches.html (last accessed May 12, 2014).

6. Winne, xvi–xvii.

7. The reporting on Huntington's health problems and the quotes have been gleaned from Mike Stobbe, "West Virginia Town Called 'Unhealthiest City' in Nation," *Quad-City Times* (Davenport, IA), November 17, 2008, A1.

8. Statistics from the Los Angeles County Department of Public Health, as reported in Associated Press, "L.A. OKs Moratorium on Fast-food Restaurants," *MSNBC*, July 29, 2008, http://www.msnbc.msn.com/id/25896233/ (last accessed February 2, 2009).

9. Ibid.

10. Kim Severson, "Los Angeles Stages a Fast Food Intervention," *New York Times*, August 13, 2008, F1.

11. Data obtained from the Centers for Disease Control and Prevention's Behavioral Risk Factor Surveillance System. Obesity is defined as having a Body Mass Index (BMI) of 30 or higher.

12. Centers for Disease Control and Prevention, "Overweight and Obesity," http://www.cdc.gov/nccdphp/dnpa/obesity/childhood/index.htm, (last accessed May 10, 2009).

13. According to the National Institutes of Health, "obese" is defined as having a Body Mass Index (BMI) of 30 or greater. "Normal" weight is a BMI between 18.5 and 25.

14. Centers for Disease Control and Prevention, "Adult Obesity Facts," http://www.cdc.gov/obesity/data/adult.html (last accessed February 3, 2014).

15. Centers for Disease Control and Prevention, "Chronic Disease Prevention and Health Promotion," http://www.cdc.gov/nccdphp/publications/aag/dnpa.htm (last accessed May 10, 2009).

16. Centers for Disease Control and Prevention, "Preventing Obesity and Chronic Diseases through Good Nutrition and Physical Activity," http://www.cdc.gov/nccdphp/publications/factsheets/prevention/pdf/obesity.pdf (last accessed April 2, 2014).

17. Maring's farmers' markets have proven so popular that Kaiser Permanente created a web page for people to find their nearest hospital farmers' market: https://healthy.kaiserpermanente.org/static/health/en-us/landing_pages/farmersmarkets/index.htm. (last accessed January 26, 2014).

Also of note, Kaiser Permanente hosts another web page devoted to Maring's recipes for healthy food, http://recipe.kaiser-permanente.org/. (last accessed January 26, 2014).

The reporting of the history of Kaiser's farmers' markets and the quote by Maring are from Project for Public Spaces, "Kaiser Farmers' Markets," http://www.pps.org/blog/kaiser-farmers-markets/ (last accessed April 2, 2014).

18. Michelle D. Florence et al., "Diet Quality and Academic Performance," *Journal of School Health* 78 (2008): 212.

19. Severson, "Los Angeles Stages a Fast Food Intervention."

20. Eric Schlosser, *Fast Food Nation* (New York: Perennial, 2002), 42–46.

Chapter 3

1. http://provomayor.com/2010/07/21/what-s-that-growing-on-the-patio/.

2. Nathan Murray, in a telephone conversation with the author, January 9, 2014.

3. Nathan Murray, in an e-mail to the author, October 14, 2013.

4. Sam Penrod, "Provo City Puts Garden to Good Use," KSL-TV, July 10, 2011, http://www.ksl.com/?sid=16321964 (last accessed January 27, 2014).

5. Heather Knight, "Mayor's Agricultural Plan Soon to Bear Fruit," *San Francisco Chronicle SFGate*, March 23, 2010: http://www.sfgate.com/homeandgarden/article/Mayor-s-agriculture-plan-soon-to-bear-fruit-3195585.php (last accessed January 27, 2014).

6. The full executive directive, which was issued by San Francisco Mayor Gavin Newsom on July 9, 2009, can be viewed here: http://www.sfgov3.org/Modules/ShowDocument.aspx?documentid=74 (last accessed January 27, 2014).

7. William H. Whyte, *The Social Life of Small Urban Spaces* (New York: Project for Public Spaces, 1980), 50–53.

8. Jill Spence, in a telephone conversation with the author, January 15, 2014.

9. Jacqueline Louie, "Community Orchards: Nature's Store," *Calgary Herald*, September 30, 2011, http://www.calgaryherald.com/travel/community+orchards/5484344/story.html (last accessed January 27, 2014).

10. Interested in building your own mason bee house? You can download the City of Calgary's easy, step-by-step instructions here: http://www.calgary.ca/CSPS/Parks/Documents/Programs/Community-Orchards/mason-bee-house.pdf (last accessed January 27, 2014).

11. Worthington Resource Site, "Transitional Gardens in Worthington," http://dsmi51.wix.com/worthingtonohio#!transitional-gardens/cx84 (last accessed January 28, 2014).

12. http://dsmi51.wix.com/worthingtonohio#!serviceberry-recipe/c1jt (last accessed January 28, 2014).

13. Michael Grunwald, "Mayor Giuliani Holds a Garden Sale," *Washington Post*, May 12, 1999, A1.

14. This quote, and the information about New York's garden auction, was culled from Laura J. Lawson, *City Bountiful* (Berkeley: University of California Press, 2005), 260–63.

15. Jerry Kaufman and Martin Bailkey, "Farming Inside Cities: Entrepreneurial Urban Agriculture in the United States," Working paper, Lincoln Institute of Land Policy, 2000, 85.

16. Bacon's quote was originally recorded in Rose DeWolf, "We Look to the Future . . . And Learn from our Past," *Philadelphia Daily News*, July 24, 2000, 05.

17. For more information on the National Vacant Properties Campaign, visit http://www.vacantproperties.org (last accessed February 8, 2009).

18. John Gallagher, "Acres of Barren Blocks Offer Chance to Reinvent Detroit," *Detroit Free Press*, December 15, 2008, http://www.freep.com/article/20081215/NEWS01/812150342 (last accessed February 8, 2009).

19. For more information on land trusts and conservation opportunities, visit Land Trust Alliance, www.lta.org or The Trust for Public Land, www.tpl.org.

20. NeighborSpace, "How We Do It," http://neighbor-space.org/howwedoit.htm (last accessed January 15, 2009).

21. Kaufman and Bailkey, 30–31.

22. Luc J. A. Mougeot, *Growing Better Cities: Urban Agriculture for Sustainable Development* (Ottawa, ON: International Development Research Centre, 2006), 64.

23. Ibid, 64–65.

24. Mayor's Press Office, "Mayor Emanuel Launches New 'Farmers For Chicago' Network For Chicago Urban Farmers," City of Chicago, March 13, 2013, http://www.cityofchicago.org/city/en/depts/mayor/press_room/press_releases/2013/march_2013/mayor_emanuel_launchesnewfarmersforchicagonetworkforchicagourban.html (last accessed January 28, 2014).

25. Kathleen E. Dickhut et al., "Chicago: Eat Local Live Healthy," City of Chicago Department of Planning and Development (2006), 2.

26. Michael Thompson, in an e-mail to the author, December 28, 2013.

27. Information about the City of Chicago's honey was obtained from Veronica Hinke, "The Bee Line: The Story behind City Hall's 'Rooftop Honey,'" *Newcity Chicago*, November 07, 2006, Food & Drink section; an e-mail from Michael Thompson, beekeeper, to the author, December 30, 2008; and a conversation with City of Chicago Cultural Center staff, January 13, 2009.

28. Michael Schacker, *A Spring without Bees: How Colony Collapse Disorder Has Endangered Our Food Supply* (Guilford, CT: Lyons Press, 2008), 2.

29. Dickhut et al., 1.

30. Ibid.

Chapter 4

1. Associated Press, "Farm's Open Harvest Draws 40,000 in Colorado," *New York Times*, November 24, 2008, A14. Also from a broadcast interview of Joe Miller, "In Colorado, Veggie Giveaway Spurs Massive Response," *All Things Considered*, NPR, November 24, 2008, http://www.npr.org/templates/story/story.php?storyId=97418921 (last accessed December 5, 2013).

2. Ibid., Associated Press.

3. Ibid.

4. Agnès Varda, *The Gleaners and I* (France: Cinè-Tamaris, 2000), DVD.

5. Gail Savina, Executive Director of City Fruit, in a telephone conversation with the author, January 14, 2014.

6. Savina bristles at the term "gleaning," precisely because it connotes the gathering of scraps, leftovers, food that is unfit for one reason or another. She prefers the more general term "harvesting." But she and her organization really are gleaning. The family—like the farmer—takes what they need from their harvest, and the rest will just go to waste. City Fruit takes the food the family doesn't want; not because it is unfit, but because it is too much. There is no shame in the endeavor. But Savina's sentiment is valid. After all, Millet and Varda worked for the same cause to erase the pervasive stigma associated with gleaning.

7. City Fruit, "Urban Orchard Stewards," http://cityfruit.org/programs/orchard-stewards/ (last accessed January 19, 2014).

8. http://foodforward.org/ (last accessed January 20, 2014).

9. http://gleaninghawaii.wordpress.com/about/ (last accessed January 20, 2014).

10. http://foodforward.org/get-involved/volunteers/ (last accessed January 20, 2014).

11. Pollan, *The Omnivore's Dilemma*, 397.

12. Quotes and statistics gleaned from various pages on the SF–Marin Food Bank website: http://www.sfmfoodbank.org/. In particular, see "Food Bank Fast Facts," http://www.sfmfoodbank.org/sites/default/files/documents/NewsCenter/fastfactsupdate10_10_13.pdf (last accessed January 21, 2014). Also, Blain Johnson, Media Contact for the SF-Marin Food Bank, in a telephone conversation with the author, January 17, 2014.

13. Gleaners, "Hunger in Indiana," http://www.gleaners.org/stay-informed/hunger-in-indiana (last accessed January 21, 2014).

14. Stacie Pierce, in a telephone conversation with the author, January 28, 2009.

15. Winne, 55.

Chapter 5

1. Contrary to popular belief, folks just don't throw tomatoes at windows or people—even when a fantastic opportunity presents itself. Former Parking Manager Tom Flaherty, from the City of Davenport, Iowa, used to grow tomatoes outside his office window, free for the taking. Folks would storm into his office, enraged over a parking ticket they had just received. If there were ever a time an urban tomato would be plucked and hurled, it would be in the heat of an argument over a parking ticket. Mr. Flaherty never once had to remove tomato pulp from his face or his office windows.

2. Though commonly considered a tropical plant, the "banana" variety of passion fruit (*Passiflora mollissima*) is more vigorous and tolerant of frost than the typical commercial varieties, making this cultivar suitable to many areas in the United States.

3. Understandably, the olive oil program at UC Davis has received considerable media attention. The information gathered for this book was gleaned from the many news articles posted about the university's success. This website in particular provides a summary: http://goodlife.uc davis.edu/olive_products/ (last accessed January 1, 2014). Also, see Jim Downing, "Tasting Success: UCD Celebrates Another Year of Turning Its Olive Mess into a Moneymaker," *The Sacramento Bee*, March 20, 2008, Business section.

4. This is precisely why Ron Finley—the guerilla gardener in South Central Los Angeles—plants food along the street outside of his house. As he figures, "I can do whatever the hell I want, since this is my responsibility and I gotta maintain it. This is how I decided to maintain it." Unfortunately, the City of Los Angeles didn't agree with Finley's particular manner of maintaining "their" public space.

5. Richard Register,. *Ecocity Berkeley: Building Cities for a Healthy Future.* (Berkeley: North Atlantic Books, 1987), 42–43.

6. Jeff Bond, "Gilman Gardens a Success; But Water Rights Remain an Issue," *Queen Anne News*, August 11, 2010.

7. If the lawns are regularly treated with chemical fertilizers and pesticides, consider if irrigation runoff would pose a risk to edibles. Also, it should be noted that reclaimed water is increasingly being used for

irrigation of ornamental landscapes by many municipalities, particularly in California. While there are ongoing debates over the use of reclaimed water for irrigating food crops, it is generally advised to avoid spraying edible parts of plants directly with reclaimed water.

8. Teva Dawson, in a telephone conversation with the author, November 14, 2008.

9. Susan Reimer, "Baltimore's City Hall Vegetable Garden: An Update," *The Baltimore Sun*, June 25, 2009, http://weblogs.baltimoresun.com/features/gardening/2009/06/baltimores_city_hall_vegetable.html (last accessed January 16, 2014).

10. Melissa Grim, Chief of Horticulture for the City of Baltimore, in a telephone conversation with the author, January 14, 2014.

11. Vermont State House Food Garden, "FAQs," http://vtstatehousegarden.wordpress.com/faqs/ (last accessed January 16, 2014).

12. Ibid.

13. The quotes and information for the Jamaica, Queens, community garden were obtained from Anne Raver, "Healthy Spaces, for People and the Earth," *New York Times*, November 6, 2008, D6.

Chapter 6

1. Kamloops Food Policy Council, "Kamloops Public Produce Program," http://kamloopsfoodpolicycouncil.com/programs/kamloops-public-produce-program/ (last accessed February 15, 2014).

2. Ibid.

3. Lawson, 202.

4. Mustapha Koc et al., eds., *For Hunger-Proof Cities: Sustainable Urban Food Systems* (Ottawa, ON: International Development Research Centre, 1999), 58.

5. Winne, 140.

6. Sheldon Margen and the editors of the University of California at Berkeley Wellness Letter, *The Wellness Encyclopedia of Food and Nutrition: How to Buy, Store, and Prepare Every Variety of Fresh Food* (New York: Rebus, 1992), 40.

7. Teva Dawson, in an e-mail message to the author, December 18, 2008.

8. Robert Mellinger, "Nation's Largest Public Food Forest Takes Root on Beacon Hill," *Crosscut.com*, February 16, 2012, http://crosscut.com/2012/02/16/agriculture/21892/Nations-largest-public-Food-Forest-takes-root-on-B/ (last accessed February 16, 2014).

9. Glenn Herlihy, in a telephone conversation with the author, January 8, 2014.

10. Jacqueline Cramer, in a telephone conversation with the author, January 9, 2014.

11. Mellinger.

12. Lawson, 52.

13. Ibid.

14. Finley: http://www.ted.com/talks/ron_finley_a_guerilla_gardener _in_south_central_la.html (last accessed January 23, 2014).

15. Pollan, "Farmer in Chief."

16. The Edible Schoolyard, "Mission," http://www.edibleschoolyard .org/mission-goals (last accessed May 19, 2009).

Conclusion

1. Lawson, 171.

2. www.sfvictorygardens.org (last accessed February 22, 2009).

3. Quoted from Lawson, 175. These goals and other proceedings from the National Defense Gardening Conference are summarized in US Office of Civilian Defense, *Garden for Victory: Guide for Planning the Local Victory Garden Program* (Washington, DC: US Government Printing Office, 1943).

4. Winne, 149–150.

5. Schlosser, 266.

6. Lawson, xiv.

7. Mougeot, vi.

8. Lyson, 76–77.

9. Winne, 54–55.

10. Lisa Van Cleef, "Gardening Conquers All: How to Cut Your Jail Recidivism Rates by Half," *SF Gate*, December 18, 2002, http://www.sfgate .com/cgi-bin/article.cgi?file=%2Fgate%2Farchive%2F2002%2F12%2F1 8%2Fgreeng.DTL (last accessed February 23, 2009).

11. Jane Gross, "A Jail Garden's Harvest: Hope and Redemption," *New York Times*, September 3, 1992, US section, http://www.nytimes.com/1992/09/03 /us/a-jail-garden-s-harvest-hope-and-redemption.html (last accessed January 19, 2014).

12. Winne, 62.

13. Pollan, "Farmer in Chief."

14. Marian Burros, "Obamas to Plant Vegetable Garden at White House," *New York Times*, March 20, 2009, A1.

Selected Bibliography

There are many fantastic published works on food security, urban agriculture, and food literacy, and the list seems to grow exponentially each year. Listed below are the principal books, papers, movies, and websites that are most relevant to *Public Produce*. Many have been cited in the book; others have not, but they have all greatly influenced my thinking. Website URLs are current as of April 2014.

Books

Cockrall-King, Jennifer. *Food and the City: Urban Agriculture and the New Food Revolution*. Amherst, NY: Prometheus Books, 2012.

de la Salle, Janine, and Mark Holland, eds. *Agricultural Urbanism: Handbook for Building Sustainable Food Systems in 21st Century Cities*. Winnipeg, MB: Green Frigate Books, 2010.

Elton, Sarah. *Consumed: Food for a Finite Planet*. Chicago: University of Chicago Press, 2013.

Hanson, David, and Edwin Marty. *Breaking Through Concrete: Building an Urban Farm Revival*. Berkeley: University of California Press, 2012.

Kingsolver, Barbara, Camille Kingsolver, and Steven L. Hopp. *Animal, Vegetable, Miracle: A Year of Food Life*. New York: Harper Perennial, 2008.

Koc, Mustapha, Rod McRae, Jennifer Walsh, and Luc J. A. Mougeot, eds. *For Hunger-Proof Cities: Sustainable Urban Food Systems*. Ottawa, ON: International Development Research Centre, 1999.

Lawson, Laura J. *City Bountiful: A Century of Community Gardening in America*. Berkeley: University of California Press, 2005.

Lyson, Thomas A. *Civic Agriculture: Reconnecting Farm, Food, and Community*. Medford, MA: Tufts University Press, 2004.

Mollison, Bill. *Permaculture: A Designers' Manual*. Tyalgum, Australia: Tagari Publications, 1988.

———. *Introduction to Permaculture*. Tyalgum, Australia: Tagari Publications, 1991.

Mougeot, Luc J. A. *Growing Better Cities: Urban Agriculture for Sustainable Development*. Ottawa, ON: International Development Research Centre, 2006.

Nestle, Marion. *Safe Food: Bacteria, Biotechnology, and Bioterrorism*. Berkeley: University of California Press, 2003.

———. *What to Eat*. New York: North Point Press, 2007.

Philips, April. *Designing Urban Agriculture: A Complete Guide to the Planning, Design, Construction, Maintenance and Management of Edible Landscapes*. Hoboken, NJ: John Wiley, 2013.

Pollan, Michael. *The Omnivore's Dilemma: A Natural History of Four Meals*. New York: Penguin, 2006.

———. *In Defense of Food: An Eater's Manifesto*. New York: Penguin, 2008.

Register, Richard. *Ecocity Berkeley: Building Cities for a Healthy Future*. Berkeley: North Atlantic Books, 1987.

———. *Ecocities: Rebuilding Cities in Balance with Nature*. Gabriola Island, BC: New Society Publishers, 2006.

Schacker, Michael. *A Spring without Bees: How Colony Collapse Disorder Has Endangered Our Food Supply*. Guilford, CT: Lyons Press, 2008.

Schlosser, Eric. *Fast Food Nation: The Dark Side of the All-American Meal*. New York: Perennial, 2002.

Sedgman, Elaine. *Public Produce: Growing Food in Public Spaces*. Kamloops, BC: Kamloops Food Policy Council, 2014. (Note: this book is only available at http://kamloopsfoodpolicycouncil.com/)

Winne, Mark. *Closing the Food Gap: Resetting the Table in the Land of Plenty*. Boston: Beacon Press, 2008.

Films

Varda, Agnès. *The Gleaners and I*. France: Cinè-Tamaris, 2000. DVD.

Woolf, Aaron. *King Corn*. United States: Balcony Releasing, 2007. DVD.

Papers, Reports, and Articles

Florence, Michelle D., Mark Asbridge, and Paul J. Veugelers. "Diet Quality and Academic Performance." *Journal of School Health* 78 (2008), 209–15.

Kaufman, Jerry, and Martin Bailkey. "Farming Inside Cities: Entrepreneurial Urban Agriculture in the United States." Working paper, Lincoln Institute of Land Policy, 2000.

Pirog, Rich, Timothy Van Pelt, Kamyar Enshayan, and Ellen Cook. *Food,*

Fuel, and Freeways: An Iowa perspective on how far food travels, fuel usage, and greenhouse gas emissions. Ames, IA: Leopold Center for Sustainable Agriculture, Iowa State University, 2001.

Pollan, Michael. "Farmer in Chief." *New York Times Magazine*, October 12, 2008.

Selected Internet resources promoting food awareness

Beacon Food Forest (http://www.beaconfoodforest.org/)
The website for what is (at the time of this writing) the largest public produce project in the United States.

Center for Urban Education about Sustainable Agriculture (http://cuesa .org/)
Of particular interest are the web pages under the "Eat Seasonally" tab.

Centers for Disease Control and Prevention (http://cdc.gov/)
This is an indispensable site for information on the rise of obesity, type 2 diabetes, and food-pathogen outbreaks in the United States.

City Fruit (http://cityfruit.org/)
I find City Fruit's website to be the most content-rich and graphically pleasing of any urban gleaning organization.

Fallen Fruit (http://fallenfruit.org/)
A must-see is the web page housing the dozens of neighborhood fruit tree maps.

Feeding America (formerly America's Second Harvest) (http://feeding america.org/)
The United States' leading hunger-relief charity. The information is both shocking and inspiring.

Food Politics (http://www.foodpolitics.com/)
The blog of Marion Nestle, our nation's foremost expert on food, food safety, and food politics.

Kaiser-Permanente (http://recipe.kaiser-permanente.org/)
This is a microsite maintained by Dr. Preston Maring, the physician who started the first Kaiser-Permanente farmers' market in Oakland, CA. Packed with great recipes and K-P farmers' market updates.

Kamloops Food Policy Council (http://kamloopsfoodpolicycouncil.com/)
A fantastic website detailing the innovative programs this nonprofit creates to bolster food literacy in Kamloops. Useful for any municipality.

Slow Food International (http://slowfood.com/)
The world's leading organization on the promotion of organic, sustainable, ethical, locally raised food.

The Edible Schoolyard Project (http://www.edibleschoolyard.org/)
One of the best websites devoted to teaching children about food and gardening.

US Department of Agriculture Economic Research Service (http://ers
.usda.gov/)
Quite valuable in understanding the economics of Big Ag.